Bodymapping
Acupuncture Technique

In the spirit of Master Tung

Cole Magbanua, MAcOM, LAc

Edited by Dr. Kim Thompson, PHD.

For information, contact:

Cole Magbanua MAcOM, LAc

Acupuncture Gateway

10235 NE Holladay St.

Portland, OR 97216

503-252-1731

www.acupuncture-portland.com

Acknowledgments

Dedicated to:

Leling, Candace, Nicole, Sierra, Ansel, and Lissette

with love

There are always so many influences that go into composing this type of work, that one cannot hope to credit them all. Please forgive me if I have left anyone out.

Firstly, I would like to mention that without the support of my wife Leling and children Candace, Ansel and Lissette, it would not have been possible to get this information onto paper.

Chris Brindley LMT did most of the wonderful artwork that makes these relationships come to life.

David Gonzales for the first drawings of these muscles.

The anatomical drawings of the muscular relations are inspired by Thieme's atlas of anatomy, 2006.

Jeffrey Weih PA, L.Ac., has worked with this information for some years now, and has been someone that I could bounce ideas off as they came up.

The many students that I have had over the years have helped tremendously in inspiring me to write this information down, and for shaping the way that it is being presented.

The Oregon College of Oriental Medicine for inspiring me to strike out on my own and giving me a place to teach some of these ideas.

Central City Concern for giving me an acupuncture job to practice this information on countless patients.

Dr. Richard Tan for my first exposure to distal point acupuncture and theory.

Dr. Wei Chieh Young for continuing my education along the distal acupuncture road and for his great explanations of Master Tung points.

The many teachers and colleagues that have influenced me over the years, John Blank, David Eisen, Robert Quinn, Roger Lore, Eric Stephens, Jimmy Chang, Hong Jin, Wei Li, Wing Ming, and David Frierman.

Regina Gilbert for her fantastic editing and word processing help.

All the patients over the years that have taught me what I know to be effective.

Table of Contents

About the author

Cole started learning holistic medicine in 1991. He studied with doctors from a variety of medical traditions including Chinese, Korean, Ayurvedic and Himalayan while traveling around the world. He graduated from The Oregon College of Oriental Medicine in 1997. He has worked in a busy public health clinic, private practice, and volunteer clinics refining and using the Bodymapping Acupuncture Technique during the last 20 years. He was faculty at the Oregon College of Oriental Medicine for 6 years and served as Clinic Supervisor, Herbal Dispensary Manager, and Teaching Faculty, sharing his unique style of Acupuncture. He holds a certificate in plant based nutrition from the Center for Nutrition Studies at Cornell University. He teaches seminars and gives lectures on Acupuncture, Chinese medicine, and nutrition around the world. He is currently in private practice in Portland, Oregon.

The journey of a thousand miles begins with one step.

-Lao Tzu

Imagination is more important than knowledge.

-Albert Einstein

Do what you do so well that people can't help telling others about you.

-Walt Disney

Introduction

What is Bodymapping Acupuncture Technique? Bodymapping Acupuncture Technique is a name for the anatomical correspondence I have discovered. It starts with the extremity images and then begins to relate specific anatomical locations. The scapula is related to the pelvis, and the iliac crest is treated by the spine of the scapula, irrelevant of the channels, pure anatomical relationships. I then move on from bony landmarks, like the ischial tuberosity related to the glenohumeral notch, and finally to muscle relationships.

This book is a culmination of 20 years of study and experience with the distal point method of acupuncture. There are correlations explained here that are useful for any bodyworker or therapist. The body of the text will go into detail about the most effective or easiest treatment for that particular tissue, and will have explanations of favorite techniques and points. I believe this work to be a part of the continuing understanding of how the body functions and how it maps relations and correlations.

The body has developed over millions of years for specific functions. The lower extremity muscles and bones function for mobility of the body. The upper extremity muscles and bones function for dexterity and fine motor skills. The muscles and bones are different from upper to lower body, though there are clear similarities that are useful for treatment. How these similarities are useful and relate is what will be presented on the following pages.

Cole Magbanua MAcOM, LAc

Section I: The Basics

Images and Channel Relationships

Distal point acupuncture is channel based treatment of qi and blood stagnation causing pain, numbness, tingling, etc. Treating with this approach is fairly simple if basic ideas are understood. Channel relations need to be memorized if you are going to treat with speed and effectiveness, and the images need to be a fluent visualization of the body as a whole or in part. I believe the channels to be not just lines, but bands of energetic influence, each flowing into the next and overlapping where they meet. I also believe there are layers of channels as we travel toward the center along physical structure, as in the chest and upper back. I will explain favorite relations and images. This set is by no means comprehensive, as there are many other viable images and relations for effective treatment.

Some of the images do not have exact relations, and one or both need some "stretching" to line up. It is helpful to think in terms of joints and where they relate, then figure the rest out from those locations.

Chapter 1: Images

HEAD

EXTREMITIES

FRONT

BACK

TORSO

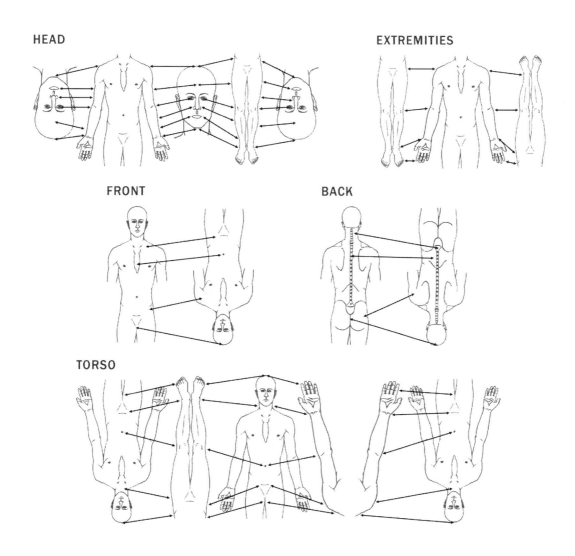

There are three images that I like for treatment. Each is used in specific ways with the channel relationship that makes it most effective.

1. Extremity
2. Torso
3. Head

Each of these images has a reversed view that can give us more points and areas to treat. Some have a front to back relationship as well. Another thing to keep in mind is that the images all work in both directions. In the head image, the ankle treats the neck (among other things), but the neck also can treat the ankle. A good example is the treatment of Achilles tendon pain.

Extremity

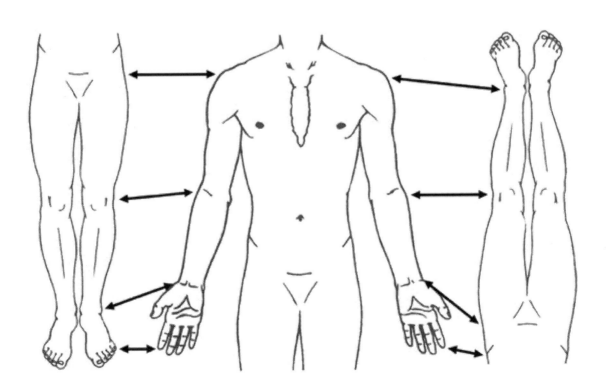

Arm – Leg

This image maps one extremity onto the other and it is very anatomical. The shoulder relates to the hip, the elbow to the knee, and the wrist to the ankle. The areas in between are related as we would expect, the upper arm to the thigh, the lower arm to the lower leg, the hand to the foot, and the fingers to the toes. Much of the basis for Bodymapping lies with this first image and the extension of it onto the torso.

There are times that I come across a difficult stagnation (like frozen shoulder) when the reversed image is less effective, and then I will use the standard relation with good results. This will typically happen toward the later treatments of a condition, where most of the stagnation is resolved, and the last 10-20% needs the more accurate anatomical equivalent to finish it off.

The reverse of this image maps the shoulder with the ankle, the elbow still with the knee, and the wrist with the hip. The reversed version is less anatomical and therefore slightly less effective, but very useful for access to difficult areas. I will often use this reversed image to treat shoulder pain using the ankle instead of the hip, and patients only need to pull up the pants leg, not pull down the pants.

The channel relationship I find most effective for these two images is the name pairs.

Needle opposite side.

Arm – Arm, Leg – Leg

Two other versions of this image map the arm or leg to themselves. The first is used in a reversed way. The hand relates with the upper shoulder, the wrist with the shoulder, the forearm with the upper arm, and the elbow with itself. The leg image is similar. The foot relates with the upper hip, the ankle with the hip, the lower leg with the thigh, and the knee with itself.

Needle same side, same channel, distally.

The second is used by needling the exact point on the opposite side. Wrist treats wrist, elbow treats elbow, etc.

Needle opposite side, same channel.

Torso

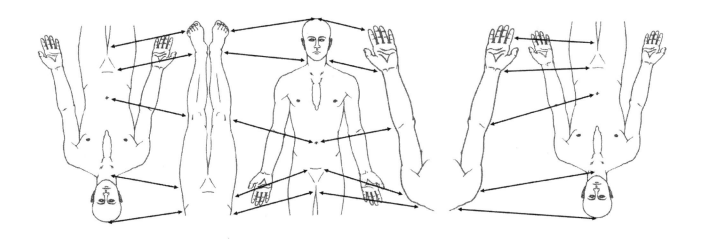

Torso – Arm, Torso – Leg

This image maps the parts of the body not covered with the extremity image. It pairs the torso (including the head), onto the arm or leg. The head relates to the hand or foot, the neck to the wrist or ankle, the chest to the forearm or lower leg, the waist/navel to the elbow or knee, the lower abdomen to the upper arm or thigh, the pelvis to the shoulder or hip, and the reproductive organs to the upper shoulder or upper hip.

The reversed version of this image flips the arm or leg over. The head relates to the upper shoulder or upper hip, the neck to the shoulder or hip, the chest to the upper arm or thigh, the waist/navel still to the elbow or knee, the lower abdomen to the forearm or lower leg, the pelvis to the wrist or ankle, and the reproductive organs to the hand or foot.

The channel relationship I find most effective for these two images is the clock opposite.

Needle opposite side.

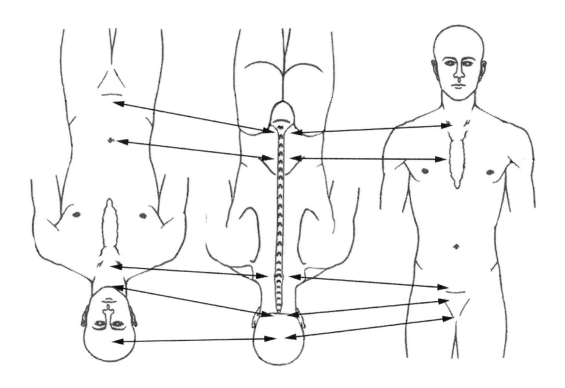

Torso, front – back, top – bottom

This version of the image maps the torso onto itself. This is simply a front to back relationship, where needling the front will treat the back, and vice versa. The spine relates to the front midline at the same level. Ribs are also treated this way by needling the same side, same rib. If the second rib is painful or effected on the right side in the back, needle near the second rib on the right side in the front.

The reversed version of this image relates the upper to lower, top to bottom. GV 20 treats GV 1, and the sternum treats the spine in the low back.

CV and GV relate well with these images, BL and KD to some degree as well, other channels relationships do not.

Torso, front – front, back – back

The second relationship is to relate the front to the front, and the back to the back, upper to lower. The best way to visualize this is to relate the bony landmarks. With this image, the sternal notch relates to the pubic symphis, the cervical vertebra relate to the sacrum, and the upper thoracic to the lumbar.

CV and GV relate well with these images, though other channel relationships do not. This relationship leads to greater understanding of the anatomical relationships on the opposite side of the torso.

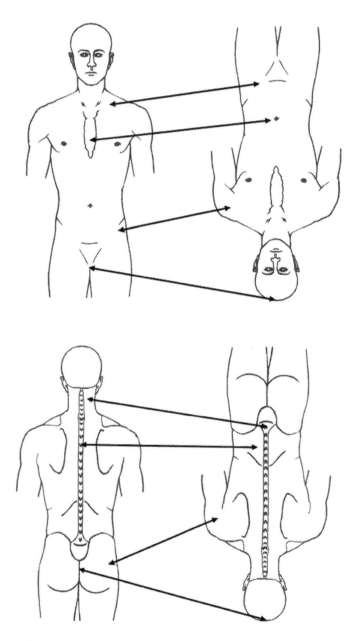

Head

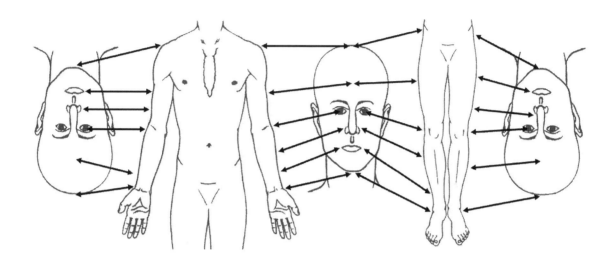

Head – Arm, Head – Leg

This image is another option for treatment of the head and maps the head onto the arm or leg. The top of the head relates to the shoulder or hip, the eye level to the elbow or knee, the nose to the radial or tibial tuberosity, the mouth to the forearm or lower leg, and the chin to the wrist or ankle.

> Think of the eye level as more of an expanded zone, a "goggle" level. Needling near the elbow or knee (SP9, ST36) will still effect the eye level.

In the reversed version of this image the top of the head relates to the wrist or ankle, the eye level still to the elbow or knee, the mouth to the upper arm or thigh, and the chin to the shoulder or hip.

The channel relationship for these images that I find most effective is again the clock opposite.

Needle opposite side.

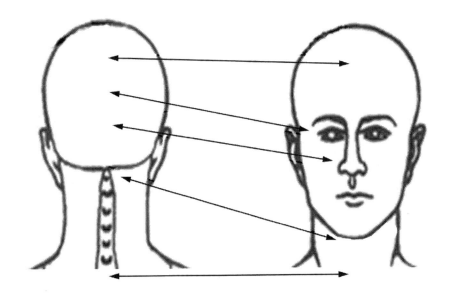

Head, front – back, top – bottom

This is similar to the torso front to back. Needle CV 24 for GV 16. Needle the external occipital protuberance (EOP) to treat the eyes. Needle GV 20 for throat problems.

CV and GV relate well with these images, as well as direct front to back.

Needle same side.

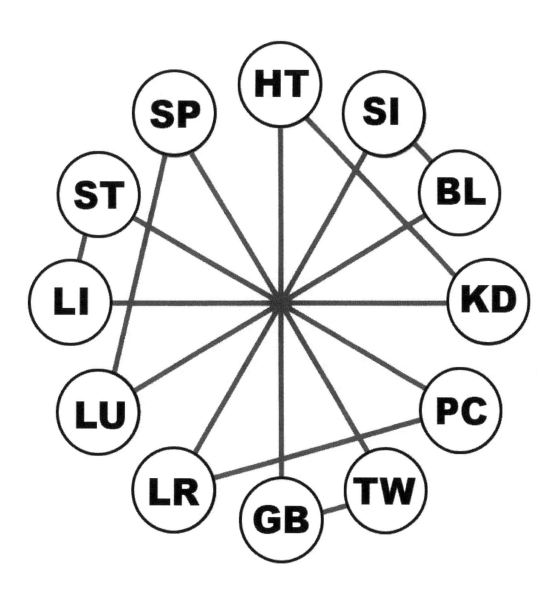

There are three main channel relations that I like and find very effective. Each has specific situations that are the most effective.

1. Name pairs

2. Clock opposite pairs

3. Same channel

The first two treat on the opposite side, while the last treats same side, and occasionally opposite side.

Name pairs

This set of channel relations is very common for most acupuncturists. It consists of the Chinese six stage names related to the channels. The two channels with the same name treat each other, opposite side. This is found most effective in the extremity images. They are often anatomically related as well.

Here is an example of a clear relation and a not so clear relation. SI3 relates with BL65 both by name pair and by anatomical location. LI4 does relate to LR3 anatomically but relates to ST43-44 by name pair. I find that the anatomical relationship is superior for clinical effectiveness.

Yang Ming	LI – ST
Shao Yang	TW – GB
Tai Yang	SI – BL
Tai Yin	LU – SP
Shao Yin	HT – KD
Jue Yin	PC – LR

Clock opposite pairs

This relationship is based on the Chinese clock, in which each channel has a designated two hour time period. This is used by pairing the channel on the opposite time of day. The time itself is unimportant, it is the energetic relationship that we can take advantage of. These are needled on the opposite side.

HT – GB

SI – LR

BL – LU

KD – LI

PC – ST

TW – SP

Same channel

This relationship is used in two ways. The first is simply a distal point down the extremity of the stagnation. Stay on the same channel, but use the images to pick the most effective point. These are needled on the same side.

The second is used on the opposite side as a mirror point. Just use the same exact point on the opposite side. This follows the anatomical relationships perfectly.

Basic Examples

Example 1: Achilles tendon pain

The Achilles tendon is between the KD and BL channels. The image that best matches is the wrist, and the name pair relationship is HT and SI. The tendon that runs between the HT and SI channels is the flexor carpi ulnaris. Needle from the SI to the HT channel under and into the tendon.

A second image is the neck related to the ankle. Needle from BL 10, traveling down the muscles on the BL channel. GV points can also be used at the same level. Try to needle between the vertebra, into the nuchal ligament.

Example 2: Upper back and shoulder pain

This is one of the most common conditions to enter the clinic. Pain and knots are often seen in muscles on trapezius, scalene, splenus, levator scapula, rhomboid, and upper ribs. Channels involved are BL, GB, SI, TW, and LI. I like the torso image with clock opposite relationships. Use LU 7-9, HT 4-7, LR 4-5, SP 5-6, KD 3-7. Opposite side and both if needed. Results should be immediate pain relief and increase in range of motion. The HT points are needled from the SI side of the ulnar tendon and threaded under the tendon perpendicularly to the HT channel.

Example 3: Ear ache

Since the ear is at both the head level and neck level, treatment often requires both images (torso and head) to be treated. The channel that travels around the ear is the TW. There is also a possibility of GB at the front of the ear and SI under and inside the ear. Treatment is usually opposite clock SP at both the ankle and knee level, SP 5,9. If the GB is involved, HT 3, and if SI is involved, LR 4,8. Since SP 5 and LR 4 are crossing points, I typically will insert 1-3 needles in the area, angling under the tibialis anterior tendon.

Section II: Comparative Anatomy

Homology of fore and hind limbs

In studying anatomy on opposite limbs, there are clear similarities and there are also differences. One of the most obvious and difficult to explain differences is with the elbow and knee. The muscles that flex the elbow do not relate to the muscles that flex the knee. At first it seems as though the theory must be flawed. On further examination of the evolution of mammals, there are some explanations.

Primitive tetrapods (four limbed vertebrates) from 360 million years ago had the basic four part limb structure humans have today.

1.   Limb girdle – shoulder or pelvis

2.   Humerus or femur

3.   Ulna (fibula) and radius (tibia)

4.   Carpals (tarsals) and phalanges

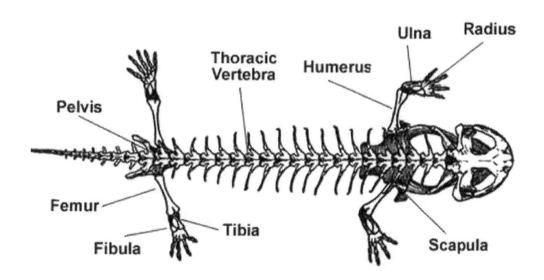

In amphibian and reptilian tetrapods, like lizards, the upper arm and leg extend nearly straight horizontal from the body, with the trunk slung between the limbs and dragging on the ground. The forearm and lower leg extend at a near right angle downward with the elbow and knee pointing outward. The weight is not centered over the limbs, but transferred outward 90 degrees. Strength is used to lift the body off the ground and there is lateral flexing of the spine when walking.

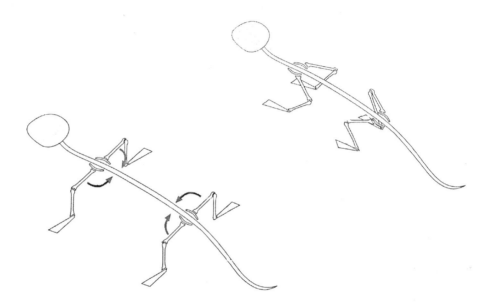

Mammalian locomotion involved a change in limb posture from sprawling to semi-erect. The limbs rotated and reoriented

Mammalian evolutionary limb rotation:

Elbow: rotation – back, rear muscle (tricep) took over extension of the elbow, the dorsal extensor became the shoulder extensor and elbow extensor.

Knee: rotation – forward, front muscle (quadracep) took over extension of the knee, the dorsal extensor became the hip flexor and knee extensor.

themselves parallel and close to the body. This provided for better balance and agility. The rear leg rotated with the knee pointing forward, and the front leg with the elbow pointing backward. In order for the palmar surfaces of the limbs to remain in contact with the ground, the forearm radius must cross over the ulna in a pronated position.

This arrangement of the structure is mostly unchanged in the human skeleton. With the lower limb rotating forward, the previous dorsal side of the limb now faces forward in a standing position. As a result, the hip flexors now also extend the knee, whereas the elbow is extended by the arm extensors.

In the lizard anatomy, the knee and elbow extensors relate, but in the human structure, with forward rotation of the knee, they no longer do. Treat with channel relationships. Use the anatomical relationships to treat the hip flexors and extensors origins, and the forearm, hand, lower leg, and foot.

Here are my thoughts on some other differences. The tibia is larger in proportion to the fibula than the radius to the ulna. This makes ST and SP channels cover more territory, as their anatomy is increased. There is also a switch of the LR and SP channels in the lower leg. SP is earth and therefor flesh, so needs to be on muscle. LR is wood and tendon/ligament, but there is not much on the inner lower leg, so it switches to the connective tissue along the tibia. In the forearm, PC travels distally between 2 tendons. GB and TW are both traveling between bones in the forearm and lower leg. When humans started becoming erect, the calf muscles enlarged, BL enlarged posteriorly taking over most of the flexion (plantar flexion) of the foot, while KD moved to the inside of the calf.

Section III: Human Anatomical Relationships

Distal point treatment and channel theory work very well together, especially when the pain is located directly on an acupuncture point. But what happens when there is a painful spot or area that falls between channels? Where exactly are the areas of influence of the channels? These questions were constantly on my mind in the early years of practice in public health. Working in public health we had lots of patients to practice on and most had some sort of pain. I was able to start mapping out where the channels of influence were by clinical experience and results.

> There are layers to the channels on the torso. The scapula and rhomboids are SI channel and treated with opposite clock LR, but the subscapularis is HT and treated by GB, and the ribs below that are GB and treated with HT, and inside the ribcage is SP and treated with TW. When looking at the chart try to think three dimensionally.

As you can see in the color chart, I have tried to keep the colors matching their 5 element relationships. Every line and area on the chart has been proven to me clinically multiple times. This chart went through 30 or more revisions before I felt like it was correct. One of the last spots to be added was the SI18 area just under the zygomatic arch. I did not include it in earlier versions of the chart because it had never presented clinically. Facial pain was always ST, LI, CV, GB, or BL. Then I had a patient with Trigeminal Neuralgia and there was one spot I just could not get to resolve. After going back to the classical charts SI18 was the exact point she was pointing to as the last spot of pain. I had completely forgotten about it because it had never come up and therefor didn't believe in its existence. In going through the images and channel relationships, I came to a tender spot on the foot between LR4 and LR3. The effect was immediate. She only needed 2-3 treatments after that point for completion of treatment and lasting relief. I now believe that the SI channel travels from SI 17 into the inner ear and along the maxilla and teeth to its expression at SI 18.

Beyond the channel theory and relationships, it became evident that the effect of treatment was even greater when anatomy was taken into account. I then started trying to relate bones, joints, muscles, tendons and ligaments on opposite limbs. These relations are not the only treatment for the tissues involved, and are not always the first or most effective treatment. The understanding that comes from these relations has been invaluable for the treatments I find most effective, and may be for you as well.

For each set of muscle relationships there are summarized actions, origins, and insertions of the muscles divided into two parts; similarities and differences. There is a comment section which explains the relationships in greater detail, and lastly an acupuncture treatment section that gives specific areas to focus treatment.

The artist has drawn the muscles in such a way that the origin and insertion are visible as an outline, and the muscle belly does not detract from the view. This gives us a better view of the relationships between muscles and bony landmarks. All relations are on the opposite side unless indicated otherwise.

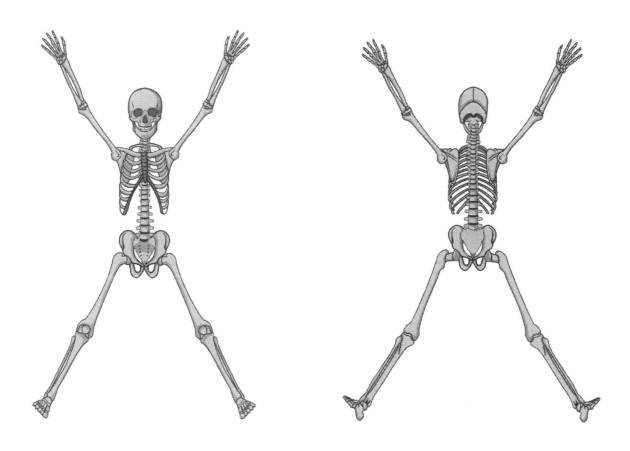

I have made the above images with the arms over the head for ease of anatomical comparison to see the opposite sided relationships. As we move from each extremity toward the body center, the relationships become clear. Initially follow the bony landmarks, then joints, and in the next chapter muscles and tendons.

Start at the extremities and move toward the body center, identifying landmarks along the way: wrist and ankle, elbow and knee, shoulder and hip. For conditions around the patella, there is no anatomical correlate at the elbow. Just follow the name pair channel relationships: LI-ST, LU-SP. It is very convenient that ST and SP are divided by the red and white skin, as LI and LU are divided by the same. The patella would be located between LU5 and LI11.

The torso gets more interesting. On the back travel from the lateral spine of the scapula and lateral iliac crest of the pelvis to the medial of both. The superior border of the scapula and the sacroiliac joint relate as well as C7-T1 and L5-S1. Move away from the center in both directions and relate sacrum and cervical vertebra, occiput/skull and coccyx. Move toward the center in both directions and relate infraglenoid tubercle and ischial tuberosity, thoracic and lumbar vertebra. On the front travel from the coracoid process and ASIS to the sternoclavicular joint/jugular notch and the pubic symphysis.

Extremities

Leg to arm

- Toes relate to fingers

- Arch relates to radial border of the first metacarpal (SP - LU)

- Foot relates to hand

- Heel (calcaneus) relates to pisiform

- Ankle relates to wrist

- Fibula relates to ulna

- Tibia relates to radius

- Tibial tuberosity relates to radial tuberosity

- Knee relates to elbow

- Femur relates to humerus

- Hip relates to shoulder

The toes and fingers are both digital hinge joints. The ankle and wrist are both complex multi bone joints. The knee and elbow are both hinge joints. The hip and shoulder are both ball and socket joints.

The long digits of the hands help with gripping and dexterity while the short digits of feet aid in balance. The big toe is in line with the other toes to ease bipedal movement while the opposable thumb of the hand is useful for gripping. The calcaneus is large for weight bearing while the pisiform is a bony attachment for the ulnar flexors. Small wrist bones improve dexterity while the ankle bones support weight. The rotational ability of the radius improves dexterity while the tibia of the leg is supportive. The olecranon at the elbow joint aids the hinge movement while the fibular head is a good attachment for the hip flexors. The patella at the knee joint aids in flexion of the knee while there is no such bone at the elbow. The trochanter on the femur creates strong weight bearing ability while the head of the humerus functions for dexterity.

Needle the opposing limb for the location given by anatomical correspondence. These are general relations, for specifics see section 3.

The base of the first metatarsal at the medial cuneiform relates to the base of the first metacarpal at the trapezium. The large area on the foot from the medial cuneiform past the navicular onto the talus at the medial maleolus relate to the smaller area on the hand from the trapezium past the scaphoid to the radial styloid process. It relates to the medial cuneiform (mid foot) but also relates to the head of the talus at the ankle.

Fingers relate to toes and hand to foot. This is basic and obvious, except for the opposable thumb. The first distal phalanx, first proximal phalanx, and first metacarpal relate as expected, but the saddle joint of the thumb at the trapezium needs multiple images. Often needles will need to be placed at SP5, and from SP5-4 to treat conditions at the base of the thumb.

Calcaneus relates to the pisiform. By following the Tai Yang and Shao Yin channels on the wrist and ankles, the anatomy is clear. This is very useful for plantar fasciitis, and other heel pain. It can even work for spur pain. The Master Tong points Mu Guan and Gu Guan are in this general location and work well for foot pain, but understanding the exact anatomy can lead to greater results. The Calcaneus is much larger than the pisiform, so the point location at the pisiform needs to be more exact, many times requiring 3 or more needles.

Knee relates to elbow and both are hinge joints. In the case of the lower and upper arm, the name pair channels have the closest relationship with the leg. Yang Ming and Tai Yin are on either side of the tibia and radius. I find that Tai Yang on the lower arm is located on the anterior and posterior sides of the ulna. The anterior (red skin, yang side) treats the channel relationships, and the posterior (white skin, yin side) treats the organ level more (LR).

Torso

- Pelvis relates to scapula

- Anterior superior iliac spine (ASIS) relates to coracoid process

- Anterior inferior iliac spine (AIIS) relates to supraglenoid tubercle

- Posterior iliac crest relates to scapular spine

- Sacroiliac joint relates to superior angle of scapula (insertion of levator scapula)

- Ischial tuberosity relates to infraglenoid tubercle

- Pubic symphis relates to sternoclavicular joint and jugular notch

- Ribs relates front to back (same side)

- Spine relates top to bottom and front to back

- Skull relates to coccyx and genitals

- Cervical vertebrae relates to sacral vertebrae

- C7-T1 relates to L5-S1

- Upper thoracic relates to lumbar

- Mid thoracic relates to lower thoracic and upper lumbar

Pelvis to Scapula

Both bones are flat and have ridges, help attach muscle from the extremity to the torso, and have ball and socket joints. When looking at the relationship of the pelvis and scapula, the sacrum relates with the inferior lateral border of the scapula. The central part of the sacrum also relates with the spine. The image works as if the scapula were fused to the spine.

To treat the SI joint requires a ligament or tendon, and the SI joint point at the wrist works very well (this is actually how this point was discovered, see section IV). Use SP5.5 and LR4.5 to treat TW15 and SI14 at the superior angle of the scapula.

Anterior superior iliac spine (ASIS) relates to coracoid process. Needle around the coracoid to treat the ASIS. For the coracoid, needle around SP5: SP-LU are name pair, ankle-shoulder are extremity image reversed.

Anterior inferior iliac spine (AIIS) relates to supraglenoid tubercle. Needle shoulder to treat hip. Use ankle to treat shoulder at ST41, extremity image reversed.

Posterior iliac crest relates to scapular spine. Needle the scapula to treat the ilium. Use BL60 area to treat the scapula.

Sacroiliac joint relates to superior angle of scapula (insertion of levator scapula). The superior angle of the scapula is the attachment of the levator scapula, a muscle, and will treat the thoracolumbar fascia.

Ischial tuberosity relates to infraglenoid tubercle. Needle insertion of the triceps long head, infraglenoid tubercle, to treat the insertion of the hamstring, ischial tuberosity. Use BL60 area to treat the opposite shoulder at SI9-10.

Ribs

Ribs relate front to back and treat themselves on the same side. First rib front treats first rib back, even if the level seems off visually. Needle close to the sternum between ribs transversely, or over the sternocostal joints.

Spine relates top to bottom

The top of the head relates to the base of the coccyx. This relation continues up and down the spine. Cervical vertebrae relate to sacral vertebrae. C7-T1 relates to L5-S1. The upper thoracic relates to the lower thoracic. The middle of the image is around T8.

Spine relates front to back

The spine relates to the midline of the torso at equal levels inferior and superior. C7-T1 relates to CV22.

The spine rotates in many directions, the sternum is static, and the linea alba is a fleshy tendon.

Some upper back pain that is not easing with regular treatments can be first or second rib issues causing the muscles around them to spasm. Ribs relate front to back (same side). Needle transverse close to the sternum or spine, between the ribs or into the ligaments around the rib attachment at the sternum.

The spine relates top to bottom and front to back. DU20 relates to DU1. The spine also relates front to back at the exact level of the spinal pain. Cervical problems can be more challenging using this method. It is possible to needle the front CV channel very superficially by tenting the skin and threading the needles along the channel over the throat area. This is uncomfortable for most patients. A better option is needling Master Tong points upright tendon on the Achilles tendon. The location of the condition will determine the depth of the needle. If the pain is along the nuchal tendon on the spine, needling into the Achilles tendon is sufficient. If the pain is on the spinous processes, the needle through the Achilles tendon needs to penetrate to the back of the tibia.

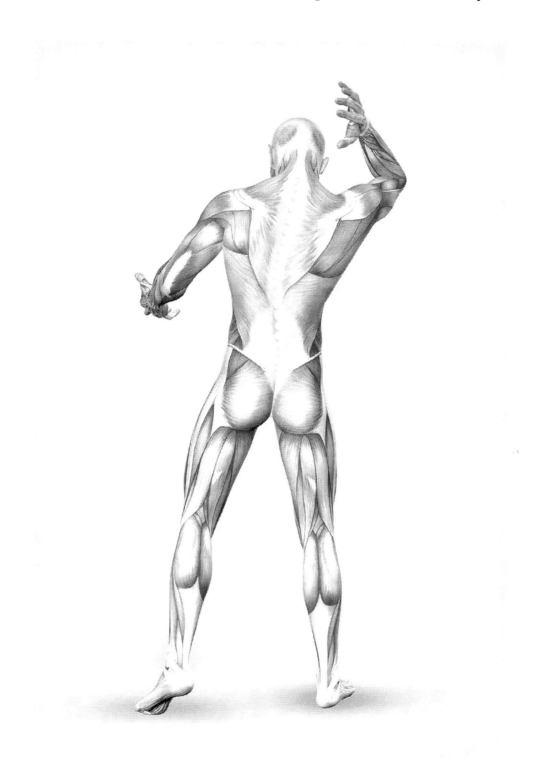

Starting at the extremities, move toward the center noticing similar muscles on opposite appendages. All the muscles around the digits and that act on the wrist/ankle and fingers/toes will relate in a very logical way. The hand extensors and the foot dorsiflexors will relate as well as the hand flexors and the foot plantar flexors. The muscles that control movement on both arm and leg flex, extend, adduct and abduct equally. There are more small bones, attachments, and muscles in the arm than in the leg which signifies the differences in use; dexterity and fine motor movement for the arm, strength, support, and mobility for the leg. Muscles around the elbow and knee relate best when the location of traditional acupuncture channels with name pairs relationship is used. Ischial tuberosity relates to infraglenoid tubercle. Which is helpful in treating triceps or hamstring insertion pain. Triceps and hamstring relate, bicep relates with some of the adductors and quadricep. Muscles that attach at the coracoid process and the ASIS relate. Bicep short head and coracobrachialis relate with tensor fascia lata. Subscapularis relates with iliacus, pectoralis minor with psoas. Subclavius relates with inguinal ligament. Teres minor relates with piriformis, gemelli and obturator. Move away from the center toward the head and genitals in both directions and relate face and genitals, eyes and testicles or ovaries, nose and penis or vagina, mouth and anus.

Extremities

- Flexor digitorum longus (leg) relates to flexor digitorum superficialis and profundus (arm)

- Extensor digitorum longus (leg) relates to extensor digitorum, extensor digiti minimi, extensor indicis (arm)

- Flexor hallucis longus relates to flexor pollicis longus

- Extensor hallucis longus relates to abductor pollicis longus, extensor pollicis longus and brevis

- Tibialis anterior relates to extensor carpi radialis longus and brevis, brachioradialis

- Tibialis posterior relates to flexor carpi radialis, palmaris longus

- Fibularis longus, brevis, and tertius relate to extensor carpi ulnaris

- Triceps surae (gastrocnemius, soleus), plantaris relate to flexor carpi ulnaris

- Supinator, pronator teres, pronator quadratus relate by location to the medial or lateral lower leg

- Biceps femoris, semimembranosus, semitendinosus, popliteus relate to triceps brachii, brachialis

- Rectus femoris insertion at tibial tuberosity relates to biceps insertion at radial tuberosity

- Vastus medialis relates to biceps brachii

- Sartorius, gracilis relate to biceps brachii

- Rectus femoris belly relates to deltoid, biceps, and brachialis

- Rectus femoris origin at asis relates to biceps brachii short head origin at coracoid process

- Vastus lateralis relates to triceps brachii lateral head, and anconeus

- Adductor longus, brevis, magnus, minimus, obturator externus, pectinius relate to pectoralis major

- Tensor fascia lata relates to biceps short head, coracobrachialis

- Gluteus maximus, minimus, medius relate to deltoidius, supraspinatus

- Piriformis, gemelli, obturator, quadratus femoris relate to teres minor, major, infraspinatus

- Supinator, pronator teres, pronator quadratus relate by location to the medial or lateral lower leg. There is not much pronation or supination of the lower leg. Treat opposite side, medial for the pronators, lateral for the supinator. Needle by channel, HT – KD, PC – LR, LU – SP. Channel treatments are great when anatomical correspondences are not available.

Torso

- Psoas relates to pectoralis minor

- Iliacus relates to subscapularis

- Inguinal ligament relates to subclavius

- Mastoid, temporalis, scalene, sternocleidomastoid (scm), splenis capitis and cervicis, trapezius, levator scapulae, rhomboid, latissimus dorsi, paraspinal, serratus, abdominis, obliques, quadratus lumborum, and others are all treated by channel and image as in section 1.

Chapter 3: Major Muscle Correlations

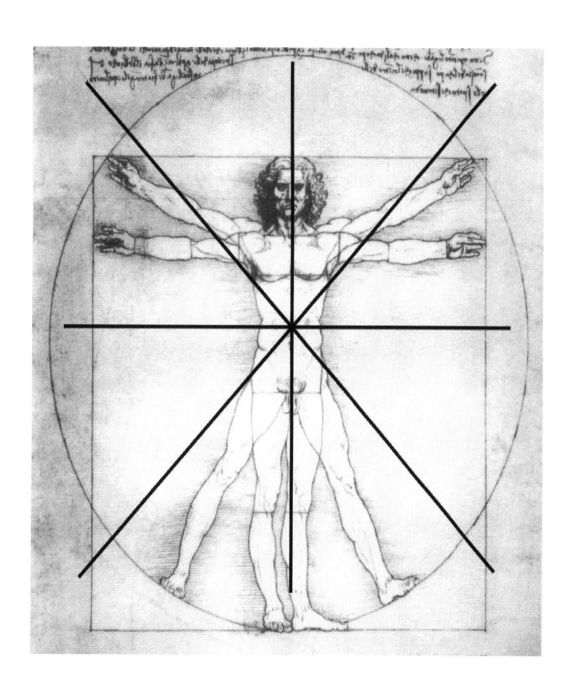

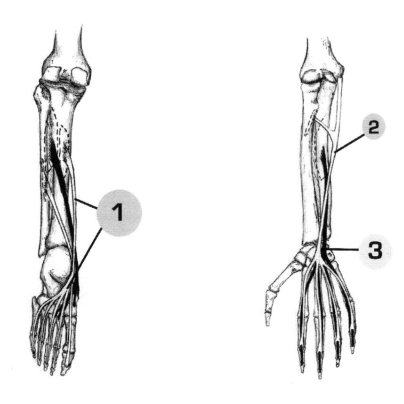

Flexor digitorum longus(1) (leg) relates to flexor digitorum superficialis(2), profundus(3) (arm)

Similarities: All muscles flex the wrist or ankle, fingers or toes.

Differences: Flexor digitorum superficialis (arm) weakly flexes the elbow. Flexor digitorum longus (leg) inverts the foot.

Comments: Flexor digitorum longus (leg) is deep to larger muscles, and difficult to access at all areas. Medial palpation and treatment is best, while the arm muscles are easier to palpate. These muscles relate by action, insertion area, and location.

Needle along HT – KD, and down into foot or hand following the anatomy. Finger and toe treatment work well with anatomical relations. Needle medial for medial and lateral for lateral.

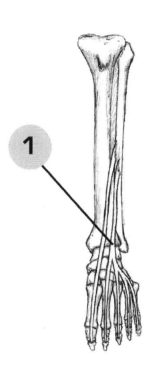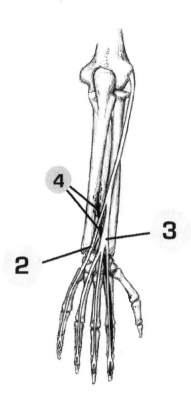

Extensor digitorum longus(1) (leg) relates to extensor digitorum(3), extensor digiti minimi(2), extensor indicis(4) (arm)

Similarities: All muscles perform extension of the wrist or ankle (dorsiflexion) and fingers or toes.

Differences: Extensor digitorum (arm) abducts the fingers, extensor digiti minimi abducts the hand (ulnar) and fifth digit. Extensor digitorum longus (leg) pronates the foot.

Comments: These muscles have similar anatomy, and treat each other well. The fact that there are more muscles in the arm for a similar function is what makes the hand and arm better suited for small movements and dexterity, and the foot and leg better for mobility and strength.

Needle by location and by channel. ST – LI, GB – TW. Fingers and toes treat each other as well, and often it is not necessary to needle the length of a digit for good results. Needling the base points of a digit (ba xie, ba feng) are often effective for treatment of the entire digit.

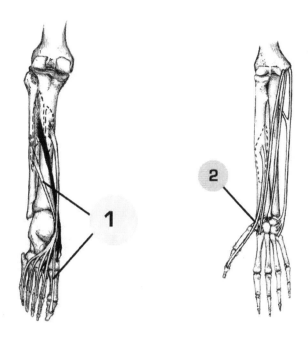

Flexor hallucis longus(1) relates to flexor pollicis longus(2)

Similarities: Both muscles flex the hand or foot, big toe or thumb, and radially deviate or supinate (invert) the hand or foot.

Differences: Flexor hallucis longus supports the medial longitudinal arch of the foot.

Comments: These treat each other well. Thumb for big toe. They relate at the wrist and ankle, but as the big toe at the foot attaches like the other toes, and is not opposable, there is a slight variation. The base of the first metatarsal at the medial cuneiform relates to the base of the first metacarpal at the trapezium. The large area on the foot from the medial cuneiform past the navicular onto the talus at the medial malleolus relate to the smaller area on the hand from the trapezium past the scaphoid to the radial styloid process.

LU 9 relates to SP 5; KD 2 – SP 4 – SP 3 relate to LU 10.

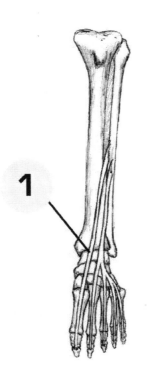 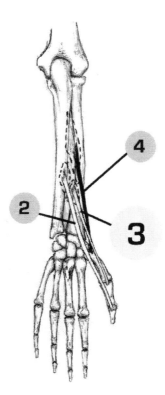

Extensor hallucis longus(1) relates to extensor pollicis longus(2) brevis(3), abductor pollicis longus(4)

Similarities: Extensor pollicis longus and extensor hallucis longus both extend (or dorsiflex) the ankle or wrist. All muscles radially deviate or invert the hand or foot. Extensor policis longus, brevis, and extensor hallucis longus all extend the big toe or thumb.

Differences: Abductor pollicis longus abducts the thumb.

Comments: The many muscles that move the thumb are limited in the foot for the big toe (not opposable). All originate from the interosseous membrane, which helps us understand how to treat them deeply.

We have an easier time treating these tendons, we can needle into, under and around them. You may not be on traditional points or channels, just follow the anatomy. This is effective for trigger finger or Dupuytren's contracture as well. We are mostly on LI – ST but also TW – GB and LU – SP or LR (here the anatomy varies from the channel relations so go by the anatomy).

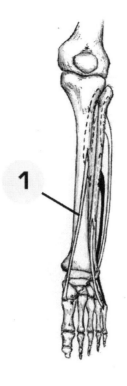 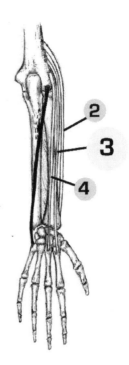

Tibialis anterior(1) relates to brachioradialis(1), extensor carpi radialis longus(3) and brevis(4)

Similarities: Extensor carpi radialis longus and brevis extend the wrist, and tibialis anterior extends the ankle (dorsiflexion).

Differences: Extensor carpi radialis longus, brevis, and brachioradialis flex the elbow. Extensor carpi radialis longus and brevis radially deviate the hand, while brachioradialis semipronates the forearm. Tibialis anterior supinates the foot.

Comments: These are the hand and foot extensors that do not act on the fingers or toes. Actions and locations are similar.

Needle by location and by channel.

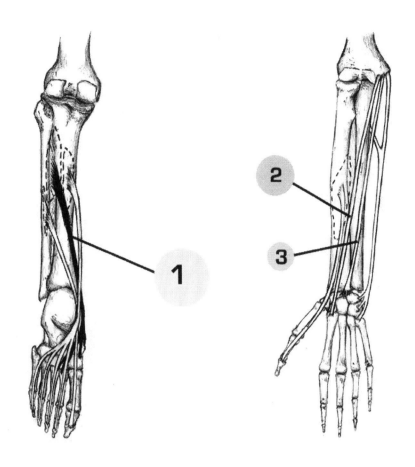

Tibialis posterior(1) relates to flexor carpi radialis(2), palmaris longus(3)

Similarities: All muscles perform flexion of the hand or foot (plantar flexion). Flexor carpi radialis and tibialis posterior both radially deviate or supinate (invert) the hand or foot.

Differences: Palmaris longus flexes the elbow.

Comments: These relate by action and location.

Treat by channel and location. BL – SI, HT – KD, PC – LR.

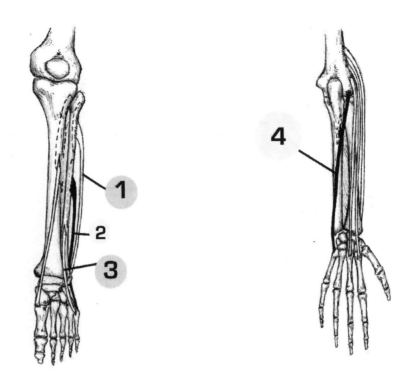

Fibularis longus(1), brevis(2), and tertius(3) relate to extensor carpi ulnaris(4)

Similarities: Extensor carpi ulnaris and fibularis tertius extend and deviate (ulnar and eversion) the hand or foot. Fibularis longus and brevis also evert the foot.

Differences: Fibularis longus and brevis perform flexion (plantar).

Comments: Fibularis tertius has the same functions and insertion as extensor carpi ulnaris, but different origins. Treat one for the other. For the origin of extensor carpi ulnaris at the lateral epicondyle of the humerus, treat from the head of the fibula toward the lateral condyle of the femur.

Needle by location and by channel. Use GB – TW to treat each other. Follow the TW channel from the wrist up to the elbow at the lateral epicondyle of the humerus, instead of the olecranon.

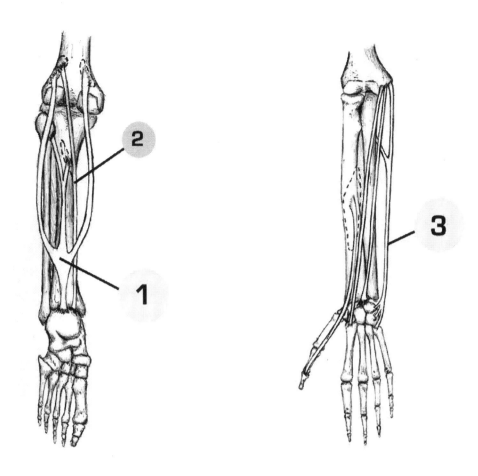

Triceps surae(1) (gastrocnemius, soleus), plantaris(2) relate to flexor carpi ulnaris(3)

Similarities: All muscles perform flexion of the hand or foot (plantar flexion).

Differences: Flexor carpi ulnaris performs ulnar deviation, while the triceps surae inverts (supinates) and flexes the knee. Plantaris plantar flexes the foot to a minor degree.

Comments: Since the pisiform and calcaneus relate, so do the insertions of the muscles onto them.

Needle BL – SI one for the other. Needling the pisiform for the calcaneus is very effective for plantar faciitis and heel pain.

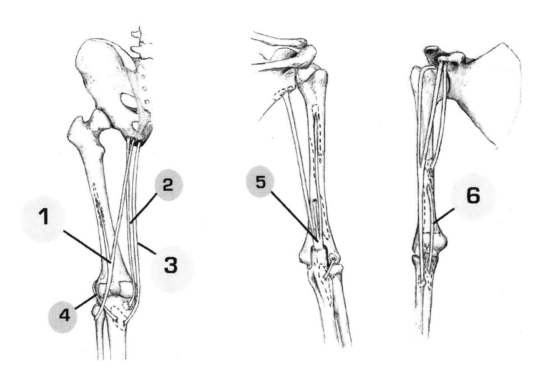

Biceps femoris(1), semimembranosus(2), semitendinosus(3), popliteus(4) relate to triceps brachii(5), brachialis(6)

Similarities: Biceps femoris, semimembranosus, semitendinosus and triceps brachii all extend the hip or arm. All leg muscles flex the knee, and brachialis flexes the elbow.

Differences: Triceps brachii extends the elbow and adducts the arm (long head). Biceps femoris externally rotates the knee, while semimembranosus, semitendinosus, and popliteus internally rotate the knee.

Comments: Triceps brachii and the hamstrings treat each other very well. The origins treat each other as well. The infraglenoid tubercle of the scapula is locationally the same as the ischial tuberosity. Brachialis relates to the short head of biceps femoris in action, and relates to vastus medialis by location. For popliteus, needle SI 8 distally down the channel.

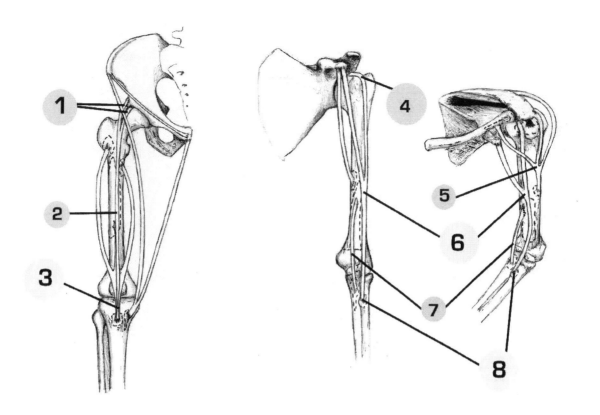

Rectus femoris insertion(3) at tibial tuberosity relates to biceps brachii insertion(8) at radial tuberosity

Similarities: Rectus femoris and biceps brachii both flex the hip or shoulder. Both insert onto the tibia or radius at a tuberosity.

Differences: Rectus femoris also extends the knee, while biceps brachii flexes the elbow, supinates the lower arm, abducts and internally rotates the upper arm.

Comments: The insertion point of biceps brachii at the lateral side of radial tuberosity is the location that is effective for treatment of tibial tuberosity. The treatment of tibial tuberosity at radial tuberosity is to needle from the outside channel near TW and threaded under the LI channel toward LU. Then along the flat of the insertion of biceps brachii at the radial tuberosity. This will take a 1.5" or more length needle. For the treatment of radial tuberosity, I will usually thread along tibial tuberosity toward pes anserinus.

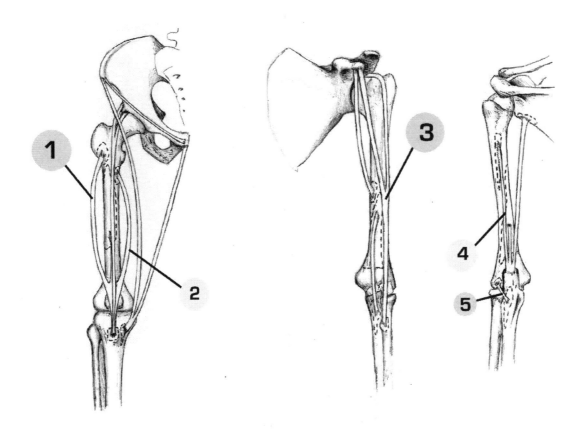

Vastus medialis(2) relates to biceps brachii(3)

Similarities: Both are located on the medial aspect of the humerus or femur.

Differences: Quadriceps femoris extend the knee, while the biceps brachii flexes the elbow.

Comments: Brachialis relates by location to vastus medialis as well. This treatment is locational, the actions are unimportant.

The channel name pair relationships work well in this case. Biceps brachii is on LU and PC channels as vastus medialis is on SP and some LR.

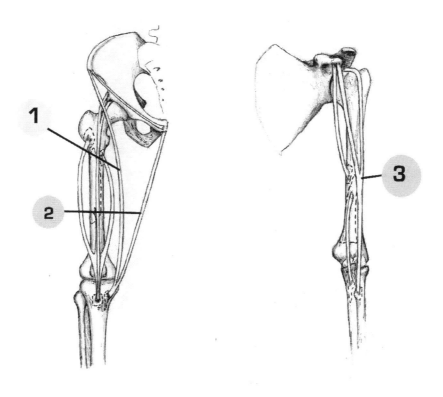

Sartorius(1), gracilis(2) relates to biceps brachii(3)

Similarities: All three muscles flex the hip, humerus, lower leg or lower arm. Sartorius and biceps brachii abduct the hip or upper arm. Sartorius and gracilis internally rotate the lower leg.

Differences: Gracilis is the only adductor. Gracilis and sartorius internally rotate the knee, while biceps supinates (externally rotates) the lower arm. Sartorius externally rotates the hip, while biceps internally rotates the upper arm.

Comments: These relationships are more by location than by action. For sartorius origin at ASIS look for treatment at the coracoid process. For gracilis origin look for treatment at the sternoclavicular joint. The belly of biceps is treated on the inner thigh along gracilis and the adductors. Biceps insertion at the radial tuberosity is treated at the tibial tuberosity and pes anserinus.

Needle as described above and match paired channels. LU – SP, PC – LR, HT – KD.

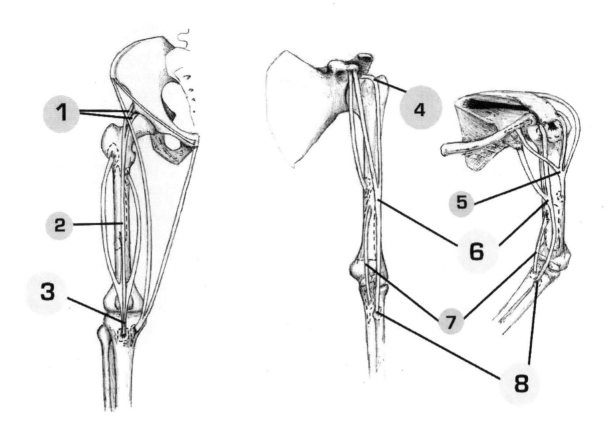

Rectus femoris belly(2) relates to deltoid(5), biceps(6), and brachialis(7)

Similarities: Rectus femoris and biceps both create flexion. All these muscles are partially in line along the anterior aspect of the leg or arm.

Differences: Deltoidius abducts and adducts, triceps extends.

Comments: The relationship of the actions of these muscles is unimportant. The anterior parts of the upper arm and leg, related locationally, are the basis for treatment.

The LI channel and ST channel are Yang Ming, needle one for the other.

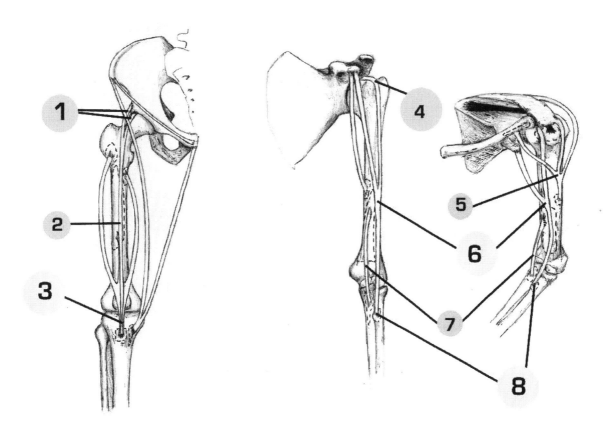

Rectus femoris origin(1) at anterior inferior iliac spine (AIIS) relates to biceps brachii long head origin(4) at supraglenoid tubercle

Similarities: Both muscles create flexion, and both are located on the anterior part of the upper arm or leg.

Differences: Rectus femoris extends the knee, while biceps flexes the elbow, supinates the lower arm, abducts and internally rotates the upper arm.

Comments: This relationship is based on the location of these muscles. The relationship is the anterior of the upper arm to thigh, and AIIS to supraglenoid tubercle.

Needle as above especially at the origins.

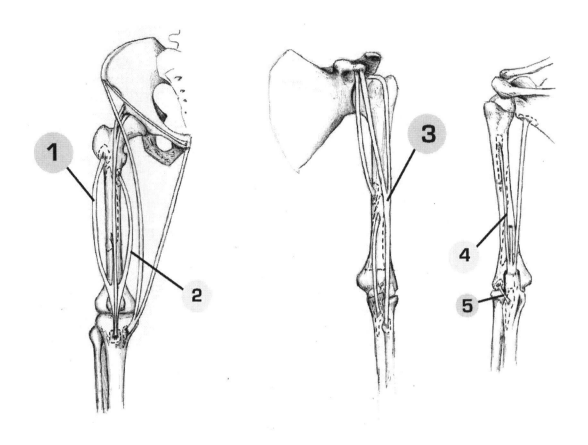

Vastus lateralis(1) relates to triceps brachii lateral head(4), anconeus(5)

Similarities: Both muscles extend the elbow or knee, and both are located on the lateral aspect of the humerus or femur.

Differences: Triceps long head moves the shoulder backward and adducts the arm.

Comments: This treatment is by anatomic location.

Triceps is located on the SI and TW channels as vastus lateralis is on the GB and ST.

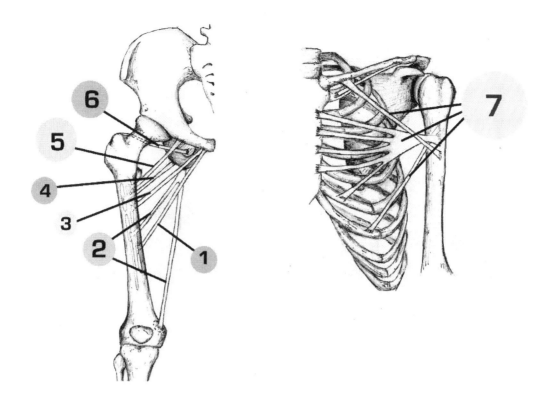

Adductor longus(1), magnus(2), brevis(3), minimus(4), pectinius(5), obturator externus(6) relate to pectoralis major(7)

Similarities: All muscles perform adduction.

Differences: Pectoralis major performs internal rotation, while adductor magnus, adductor minimus, obturator externus, and pectinius externally rotate. Adductor longus and brevis also create flexion.

Comments: This relationship is based on action, and not often used in treatment. For treating the adductor group, use anatomic imaging, and treat the upper arm around the biceps brachii, especially the pectoralis major insertion at the humerus.

The adductor group is treated by needling down the PC and LU channels on the upper arm into the biceps brachii. The pectoralis major is treated by channel, using image and channel relations, see section 1.

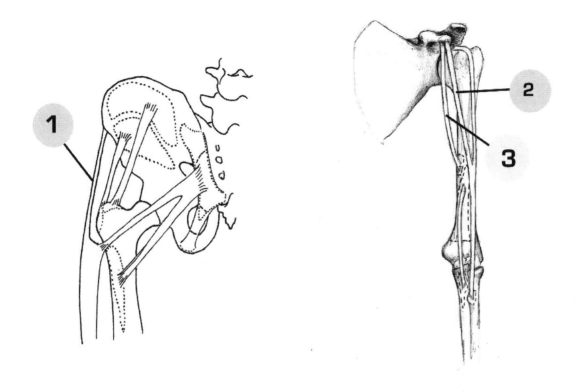

Tensor fascia lata(1) relates to biceps short head(2), coracobrachialis(3)

Similarities: TFL attaches to anterior superior iliac spine (ASIS) as biceps short head and coracobrachialis attach to coracoid process. TFL inserts into the iliotibial band, as short head biceps meets long head. TFL, biceps, and coracobrachialis all internally rotate. TFL and biceps abduct and flex.

Differences: Coracobrachialis adducts and anteverts. TFL tenses the fascia lata of the iliotibial tract.

Comments: The main relation is not in the muscles, but in the origin at ASIS and coracoid process. As the TFL runs distally toward the IT band, follow the biceps short head and coracobrachialis distally as well.

Needle coracoid process for ASIS. Needle biceps short head and coracobrachialis for TFL.

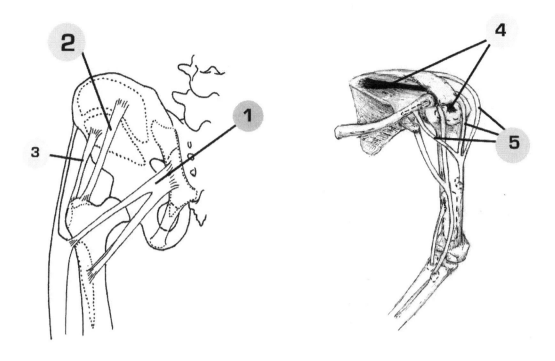

Gluteus maximus(1), gluteus medius(2), gluteus minimus(3) relate to supraspinatus(4), deltoidius(5), infraspinatus

Similarities: All the gluteus muscles extend, abduct, and externally rotate the hip. Gluteus minimus and medius also flex and internally rotate the hip. Gluteus maximus adducts the hip. Deltoidius adducts, abducts, externally rotates, and internally rotates the arm. Supraspinatus abducts the arm. Both sets of muscles surround their joints, working most of the adduction and abduction, internal and external rotation, depending on the part of the muscle used.

Differences: The deltoidius moves the shoulder and arm forward and backward (anteversion, and retroversion). The gluteus muscles stabilize the hip, which if the ilium wasn't locked at the sacroiliac joint and pubic symphis, would function to antevert and retrovert the hip.

Comments: The posterior deltoid insertion along the spine of the scapula is related to the gluteus maximus insertion along the ilium. The lateral deltoid and gluteus relate as well. The deltoid insertion on the humerus relates to the gluteus insertion into the iliotibial tract, and gluteal tuberosity. The supraspinatus relates to the gluteus medius mostly, and the gluteus minimus to a lesser extent.

I will rarely treat the upper arm with the upper leg. This is because of access. For arm symptoms I will typically reverse the image to the ankle and lower leg, keeping the name pair channel relationship, needling opposite side. The anatomy is not very accurate here and you need to let the channel be your guide. With a few stubborn frozen shoulder cases, I have needed the hip muscles to get the anatomy correct and finish off the problem, but this is typically a last resort. To treat the iliotibial tract, needle from the lateral deltoidius down the side of the arm to the insertion of the triceps onto the ulna (TW channel). The deltoidius originates in part from the clavicle which is on LU and LI channels. The gluteus muscles do not follow this origin along the front of the hip or ASIS. To treat this, just needle by channel; LI – ST, LU – SP (again I usually get this from the reversed lower leg image, see section 1).

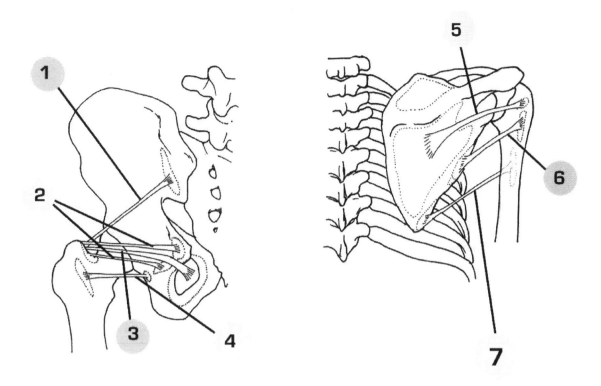

Piriformis(1), gemelli(2), obturator internus(3), quadratus femoris(4) relate to infraspinatus(5), teres minor(6), teres major(7)

Similarities: Both sets of muscles create shoulder or hip external rotation. Hip muscles run deep to gluteus muscles, and shoulder muscles are deep to deltoidius.

Differences: Teres major relates by location only, and has different actions. It adducts, internally rotates, and retroverts the arm. Some hip rotators also adduct the leg, but none internally rotate.

Comments: Teres minor treats piriformis and is the main relation. Teres Major and infraspinatus have a lesser relation.

For piriformis, needle scapula insertion for sacral insertion, muscle belly for muscle belly, and humeral insertion for trochanter insertion. To treat teres muscles and infraspinatus, I go to the opposite ankle around BL 60 – 61 and needle superficially.

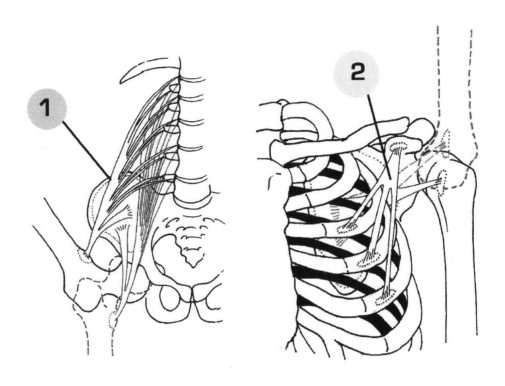

Psoas(1) relates to pectoralis minor(2)

Similarities: Both muscles are at the front of the body, and both run deep to other muscles.

Differences: Psoas attaches to the spine, flexes the hip, and externally rotates the leg. Pectoralis minor attaches to ribs and acts on the scapula, with no action on the arm.

Comments: This seems too work not from the origin, insertion or action, but these muscles are related very well on acupuncture channels, and locationally on opposite sides.

Needling the belly of the pectoralis minor seems to work best for treating the elusive psoas. Another useful point for the psoas is same side SP 5. For pectoralis minor, I will usually use insert a needle near SP 5 opposite side because the psoas is difficult to needle.

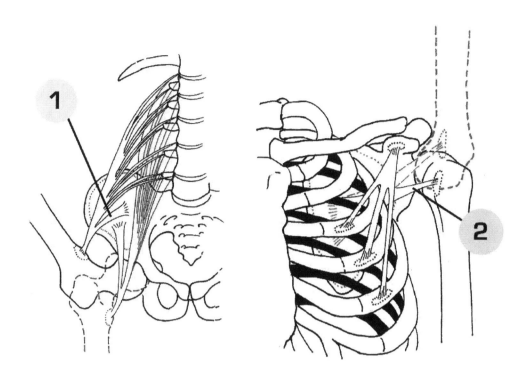

Iliacus(1) relates to subscapularis(2)

Similarities: Both originate on the flat of the pelvis or scapula, and perform internal rotation.

Differences: Iliacus joins psoas in flexion while subscapularis only internally rotates.

Comments: Both of these are hard to get to, but still have effect if treated.

Needle one to treat the other. I use other treatments for both of these muscles, though the relationship is still important. I find that the iliacus is on the belt channel and therefor use GB 41 on the same side. For the subscapularis, I find that it is on the HT channel, palpable from HT 1, and I treat it using opposite GB 39 area (see section 3 for specific needle technique).

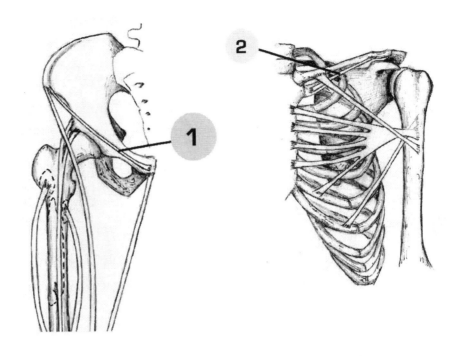

Inguinal ligament(1) relates to subclavius(2)

Similarities: Both are toward the front of the torso, small in nature, and travel transversely.

Differences: The inguinal ligament attaches from the anterior superior iliac spine (ASIS) to the pubic tubercle, and has no specific action. The subclavius originates from the first rib medially, attaches to the lateral inferior clavicle, and has a steadying function on the clavicle.

Comments: These are related locationally, and not by function. The subclavius is used to treat the inguinal ligament, which when tight or symptomatic can cause low back, hip tightness, nerve impingements, circulation issues in the leg, or reproductive problems.

Bodymapping Acupuncture Technique

I very rarely find symptoms with the subclavius, though the inguinal ligament is often tender with hip or low back issues. This relationship makes the treatment of the inguinal ligament easy. Needle along the inferior side of the clavicle transversely, laterally, and in an upward direction into the subclavius muscle, between the first rib and the clavicle, being careful of the lung and the brachial plexus.

Section IV: Strategies and Favorite Points

This list of points are the most effective and most used in our clinical practice. We are including indications, locations, special needling instructions, imaging theory, and comments. It is best to see them being needled to witness the effectiveness in person and we recommend attending a live seminar for demonstrations and practice of needle location and techniques. This is especially important with the SI Jt point, HT4-7, KD27, SI9-10, radial tuberosity, glenohumeral notch, pectoralis minor, GB41, GB39, Achilles tendon, pisiform, SP5/LR4, LR3.5, KD6, KD3-7, and BL60.

When needling we find it helpful to think of the tissue we are treating and try to needle to the level of condition. Needle skin for skin, muscle for muscle, etc. Chronic conditions use longer needles, deeper insertion. For example, children often only need superficial needling and short duration. Classical functions of points are still very useable and not included here.

Chapter 1: Points list

LU1-2

Indications: Pain and tenderness at the ASIS (anterior superior iliac spine), TFL (tensor fascia lata) pain or tenderness, psoas pain.

Location: This zone is located at the traditional location, and encompasses an area from LU1-2 extending down the short head of the biceps.

Needling information: Needle perpendicularly, 0.5-1.0 cun in depth. Contralateral.

Imaging: Torso image – torso treats itself top to bottom.

Comments: The coracoid process is anatomically equivalent to the ASIS. The TFL is related with the short head of biceps or coracobrachialis. Use 2-3 needles to cover the area. Needling further down onto pectoralis minor will treat psoas very effectively.

Case Study: Pg. 132, 148.

LU5-6

Indications:

1. BL channel quadratus lumborum muscle tension and pain, upper lumbar or lower thoracic pain, BL channel.

2. BL channel headache at eye level, eye pain at BL1-2.

3. Knee pain at the pes anserinus (SP channel).

Location: This zone is located at the traditional location, and encompasses an area from LU5-6.

Needling information:

1-2. Needle perpendicularly, 0.5-1.0 cun in depth. Contralateral.

3. Needle deeply from the LI or TW channels under the radialis muscles medially passing through the attachment of the biceps tendon at the radial tuberosity. 1.0-2.0 cun in depth. Contralateral.

Imaging: LU is opposite clock with BL.

1. Torso image – elbow is located at the navel.

2. Head image – elbow is located at eye level, all around the head.

3. Extremity image – elbow is located at knee level.

Comments:

1. Use 1-3 needles to cover the area. Used in conjunction with BL58 zone and the Ling Gu set for spinal pain as well.

2. This point can also help if the headache is on or close to the GV channel. The image is expanded 2 or more inches above and below the eyes. Will not treat BL channel on the top of the head or at the base of the occiput. LU10 contralateral is a good additional point if LU5 does not relieve the pain.

3. While looking for a way to treat knee pain at the insertion area of the pes anserinus

and studying the anatomy of the forearm, it became clear that needling the insertion of the biceps at the radial tuberosity would be useful. A perpendicular insertion from LU5 area just gets a small portion of the insertion, but if needled from the lateral side, the point can penetrate medially across the insertion.

Case Study: Pg. 121, 127, 128, 137, 145.

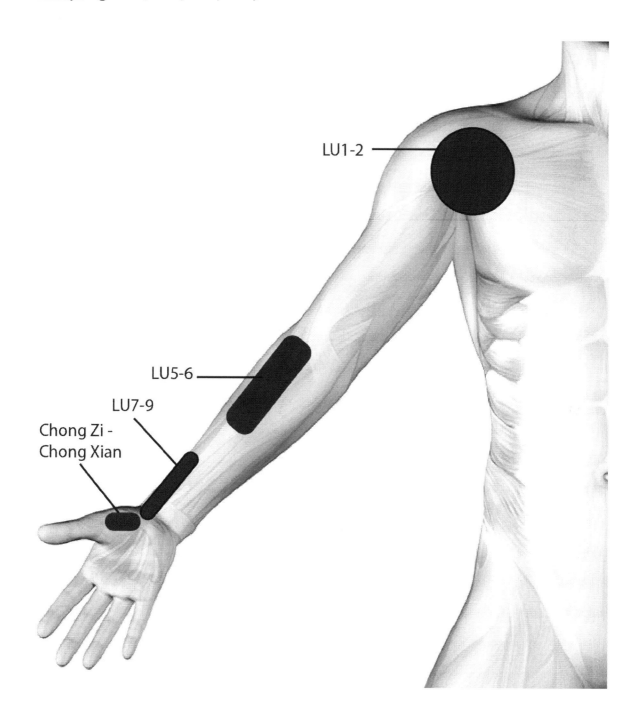

LU1-2

LU5-6

LU7-9

Chong Zi – Chong Xian

LU7-9

Indications:

1. Vertex headache on BL channel, occipital headache on BL channel.

2. BL channel neck pain and conditions BL10-11 area, base of skull to T1 level.

Location: This zone is located at the traditional location, and encompasses an area from LU7-9.

Needling information: Needle from medial side, tenting and threading the needle distally along the channel. 0.25-1.0 cun in depth transversely. Contralateral. As many as 4 needles may be needed if the entire area of the neck is involved.

Imaging: LU is opposite clock with BL.

1. Head image – wrist is located at the top of the head. Torso image – wrist is located at the base of the skull.

2. Torso image – wrist is located at the base of the skull. LU7 is the location of about T1.

Comments:

1. This point can be needled from LU8 threading into LU9 for greater effect. Pinching the skin up or "tenting" while needling makes the threading easier. If the headache is located higher on the occiput near the external occipital protuberance, and still on the BL channel, needle further distal on the LU channel toward LU10.

This point can also help if the pain is on GV channel. True GV channel headaches are rare, most are referring from BL channel.

2. This point can be needled from LU7 threading into LU9 for greater effect. This point can also help if the pain is on GV channel.

Case Study: Pg. 122, 124, 138, 141, 142, 143, 151.

Chong Zi – Chong Xian

Indications: Rhomboid pain, upper back pain.

Location: This zone is located 0.5 cun on either side of LU10 on the thenar eminence.

Needling information: Needle perpendicularly, 0.5-1.0 cun in depth. Contralateral.

Imaging: I believe this area to be a lung reflex. In the SU JOK system of Korean hand acupuncture, this area is lung. Master Tung also has this area as related to the lung on his palmar system.

Comments: These are great Master Tung points that are very effective at treating rhomboid pain especially when there are veins and/or a history of lung problems. These can also be bled for the most severe cases.

Case Study: Pg. 126, 143.

Ling Gu

Indications: Low back pain and sciatica.

Location: Proximal to LI4, just distal to the junction of the first two metacarpals.

Needling information: Needle perpendicularly, 0.5-1.0 cun in depth. Contralateral.

Imaging: Torso image – wrist relates to L5-S1, hand relates to sacrum and genitals.

Comments: This point is used with Da Bai, SI3,4, and SI Jt pt when needed.

Case Study: Pg. 128, 130, 146, 146.

Da Bai

Indications: Low back pain and sciatica, assistant to Ling Gu.

Location: Located at LI3.

Needling information: Needle perpendicularly, 0.5-1.0 cun in depth. Contralateral.

Imaging: Torso image – wrist relates to L5-S1, hand relates to sacrum and genitals.

Comments: This point is used with Ling Gu, SI3,4, and SI Jt pt when needed.

Case Study: Pg. 128, 130, 146, 146.

LI5

Indications: Sore throat of any kind.

Location: This point is located in the classical location.

Needling information: Needle perpendicularly, 0.5-1.0 cun in depth. Contralateral or ipsilateral.

Imaging: Torso image – the base of the neck is located at the wrist. LI treats itself, and LI is name pair with ST.

Comments: This point is needled from distal toward proximal, or from proximal toward distal. The wrist crease is the base of the chin and top of the throat. The closer to LI5, the higher up the throat the point treats. This point treats both channels around the throat, LI and ST. If the condition is central and on the CV channel, needle both sides. Very rare CV channel cases will need the GV needled on the cervical vertebra to effect relief.

Case Study: Pg. 125, 141.

LI6-8

Indications: Chest pain on KD or ST channels.

Location: This zone is located at the traditional location, and encompasses an area from LI6-8.

Needling information: Needle obliquely, 0.5-1.5 cun in depth. Contralateral.

Imaging: Torso image – forearm is located at the chest. LI is opposite clock with KD, LI is name pair with ST.

Comments: Thread the needle along LI channel. LI treats both KD and ST and covers a large area of the chest. Tent the skin up to thread the needles along the channel. Use in conjunction with PC5-6 which will treat ST and PC channels. With these 2 zones the entire chest is covered.

Case Study: Pg. 131, 148.

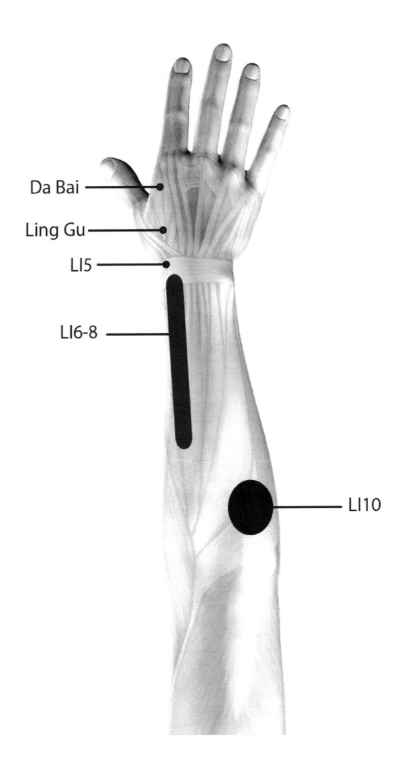

Da Bai

Ling Gu

LI5

LI6-8

LI10

LI10

<u>Indications:</u> Hara zone: lung area lower right quadrant.

<u>Location:</u> This point is a zone located from classical LI10 toward the TW channel.

<u>Needling information:</u> Needle perpendicularly, 0.5-1.0 cun in depth.

<u>Imaging:</u> Torso Image – the elbow is located at the navel level. TW treats SP with opposite clock. Contralateral.

<u>Comments:</u> For hara release of lung zone: lung area in lower right quadrant. Use 1-2 needles. This zone is located at the appendix, which is mostly lymph tissue and occupied by massive amounts of beneficial gut bacteria. This storehouse of bacteria is used to repopulate the gut in the case of infection or in modern times antibiotics. There has been a large amount of recent research on the role of the gut flora and its importance in the immune function, a fact that Chinese medicine has been treating for thousands of years. Since the lungs in Chinese medicine are the seat of the immune system, this area is a lung zone in the aspect of the immune function.

<u>Case Study:</u> Pg. 134, 140.

ST32

Indications: Chest pain, physical heart problems.

Location: This zone is located at the traditional location, and encompasses an area from 1 cun below ST32 proximally to mid thigh along the ST channel.

Needling information: Needle perpendicularly, 1.0-1.5 cun in depth. Ipsilateral.

Imaging: Torso image – thigh is located at the chest. ST treats itself.

Comments: These are great Master Tong points called Tong Guan, Tong Shan, and Tong Tian, and are usually needled with 2-3 points.

Case Study: Pg. 132, 149.

ST36-37

Indications:

1. Bell's palsy, facial paralysis.
2. Hara zones: large intestine area right or left.

Location: This point is a zone located from ST36-41 in the classical location.

Needling information: Needle perpendicularly, 1.0-1.5 cun in depth. Ipsilateral.

Imaging: ST treats itself with same channel. Ipsilateral.

1. Head image – the eye is located at the knee, and the eye to mouth area is located at the lower leg.

2. Torso Image – the knee is located at the navel level.

Comments:

1. Bleed ST channel at the shin for blood stagnation and wind, the main causes of bell's palsy. I often prick these points with a lancet or three edged needle and use a disposable suction cup to increase the blood flow.

2. For hara release of large intestine zones: large intestine area right - ST36-36 ipsilateral, large intestine area left quadrant - ST36-37 ipsilateral.

Case Study: Pg. 134, 137, 140, 141, 147, 149.ST38-39

Indications: Breast pain on sides of breasts, breast lumps, breast fibroids, breast tenderness with menstruation.

Location: This zone is located at the traditional location, and encompasses an area from ST38 distally 3 cun along the ST channel.

Needling information: Needle perpendicularly, 1.0-1.5 cun in depth. Contralateral or ipsilateral.

Imaging: Torso image – lower leg is located at the chest. ST is opposite clock with PC. ST treats itself.

Comments: Needle from ST38-41. When patients present with breast tenderness or pain, I always ask them to palpate and tell me if they feel the tenderness from the side of the breast at PC channel or more frontal at the nipple line on ST channel. Needle ipsilateral for ST channel and contralateral for PC. Use this point in conjunction with PC5-6.

Case Study: Pg. 132, 141, 149.

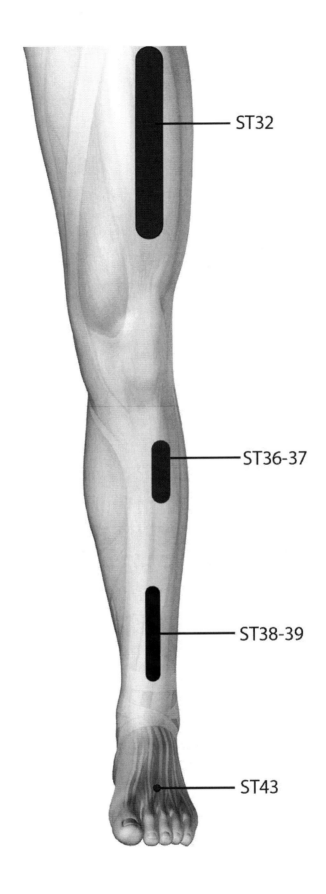

ST32

ST36-37

ST38-39

ST43

Bodymapping Acupuncture Technique

ST43

Indications: Tooth pain at the LI channel

Location: This point is located at the classical location.

Needling information: Needle perpendicularly, 0.5-1.0 cun in depth. Contralateral or ipsilateral.

Imaging: Torso image – the head is located at the foot. ST treats itself with same channel ipsilateral, and treats LI with name pair contralateral.

Comments: The upper teeth on the maxilla are LI channel, and treated contralateral. The lower teeth on the mandible are ST channel and treated ipsilateral. Treat in conjunction with LI points.

Case Study: Pg. 140.

SP5/LR4

Indications:

1. SI17 or TW16-17 area pain at corner of jaw, scalene muscle pain at the TW or SI channels.

2. Ear pain and problems at the neck level, ear infection.

3. LU1-2 area pain.

4. Hara zones: liver right or left side.

Location: This point is an area of both the LR4 and SP5 classical locations.

<u>Needling information:</u> Needle perpendicularly toward ST41, 0.5-1.5 cun in depth. Contralateral. Thread under the tibialis anterior tendon.

<u>Imaging:</u>

1-2. Torso image – the base of the head is located at the ankle. LR is opposite clock with SI, SP is opposite clock with TW.

3. Extremity image – the ankle is located at the shoulder. SP is name pair with LU.

4. Torso image – the base of the trunk is located at the ankle.

<u>Comments:</u> This point is in an area that I believe is a true crossing zone, where LR and SP merge. Insert 1-3 needles in this area.

1. It is good at treating corner of the jaw pain. It treats the scalene muscles on the TW and SI channels.

2. This point is good for ear pain or infection in conjunction with SP9. The ear is at the level of the eye and at the level of the base of the skull at the same time. Two images are needed for these areas. Eye level at the knee with head image and base of skull level at the ankle with torso image.

3. This point works well for front shoulder pain on the LU channel. It will treat the coracoid process and the muscle attachments there; biceps short head, pectoralis minor, and coracobrachialis. If needled deeply through to ST41, LI channel at the shoulder is treated as well.

4. For hara release of liver zones: liver area upper right quadrant - LR4 ipsilateral, liver area lower left quadrant - LR4 ipsilateral.

<u>Case Study:</u> Pg. 35, 37, 71, 124, 132, 138, 139, 144, 147, 152.

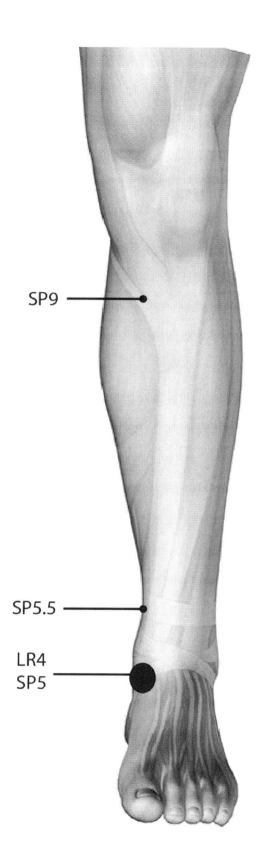

SP9

SP5.5

LR4
SP5

SP5.5

Indications: Levator scapula muscle insertion pain at the superior angle of the scapula.

Location: This point is located between 1 and 2 cun distal to SP6.

Needling information: Needle perpendicularly 0.5-1.5 cun in depth. Contralateral.

Imaging: Torso image – the neck is located at the ankle, upper back at the lower leg. SP is opposite clock with TW.

Comments: This point can take 1-3 needles and releases that knot that everyone has at the levator scapula insertion. The levator insertion is actually located at SI14, which should need a LR pt to treat it (contralateral), but SP5.5 works better. This means that either the levator insertion is located at a TW point, or that SP5.5 is also a LR point. I tend to think of the levator insertion as TW because TW5 (ipsilateral) can sometimes help as well. It could be that TW and SI overlap here like SP5 and LR4 may overlap. Usually painful areas that have overlapping channels require more than 1 channel to treat them (see low back 12th rib).

Case Study: Pg. 126, 138, 141, 142, 143.

SP9

Indications:

1. TW channel headache, temple headache, ear problems.
2. Hara zones: spleen area central or left.

Location: This point is located at the traditional location.

Needling information: Needle perpendicularly, 1.0-1.5 cun in depth. Contralateral.

Imaging:

1. Head image – knee is located at eye level, all around the head. SP is opposite clock with TW.

2. Torso image – knee is located at navel level. SP treats itself.

Comments:

1. Some headaches are described as behind the eye. I always ask the patient if it feels more behind BL1, GB1, or from the side at the temple. Many times it is located from the temple. We often see in clinic that temple headaches come on after eating badly, and at the seasonal change of summer to fall. Occasionally they are related to jaw or tooth pain, and those will need to be addressed for relief.

2. For hara release of spleen zones: spleen area upper left quadrant - SP9 ipsilateral, spleen area center - SP9 either side or bilateral. The upper left SP zone is often seen with pancreatic problems.

Case Study: Pg. 122, 134, 139, 147.

HT3

Indications:

1. GB channel headache at eye level, eye pain at GB1.

2. GB2 pain, joint popping or temporalis muscle pain.

3. Lower rib and flank pain. Herpes zoster or shingles on GB channel.

Location: This point is located closer to PC3 than the traditional HT3, look for a painful gummy location.

Needling information: Needle perpendicularly, 0.5-1.0 cun in depth. Contralateral.

Imaging: Head image – elbow is located at eye level, all around the head. Torso image – elbow is located at navel level. HT is opposite clock with GB.

Comments:

1. The image is expanded 2 or more inches above and below the eyes. Will not treat GB channel on the top of the head or at the base of the occiput. HT8 contralateral is a good point if HT3 does not relieve the pain.

2. This point treats all GB areas around the TMJ. Since the point is located at a joint, it will treat the joint as well as the muscles attaching around the joint.

3. Lower rib pain is very common with herpes zoster or shingles. It can manifest anywhere, but most are on the hypochondriac area. GB is just one channel that is typically involved, and others will need treatment as well.

Case Study: Pg. 121, 122, 127, 137, 138, 150.

HT4-7

Indications:

1. Vertex headache on GB channel, occipital headache on GB channel.

2. GB channel neck pain and conditions from the base of skull to T1 level.

3. Achilles tendon pain and tightness.

Location: This zone is located on the lateral side of the flexor carpi ulnaris. From 0.5 to 1.5 cun proximal to the pisiform.

Needling information: 0.5-1.2 cun in depth. Contralateral.

1. Needle from lateral side under ulnar tendon, distally angled toward traditional HT7.

2-3. Needle from lateral side under ulnar tendon, toward the traditional HT channel.

Imaging:

1. Head image – wrist is located at the top of the head. Torso image – wrist is located at the base of the skull. HT is opposite clock with GB.

2. Torso image – the wrist crease is located at the base of the skull. HT7 is at GB20 level, and HT 4 is at T1 level. HT is opposite clock with GB.

3. Extremity image – wrist is located at the level of ankle.

<u>Comments:</u>

1. Getting the angle correct of this point is key for its success. If the headache is located higher on the occiput near the external occipital protuberance, and still on the GB channel, needle further up the pisiform from HT7 on the palmar side.

2. This zone can take up to 4 needles for severe neck pain on the GB channel. Usually neck pain is on multiple channels and the LU7-9 zone is often needled along with this. It is easier to needle these points with the forearm in a prone position.

3. The Achilles tendon correlates with the tendon of flexor carpi ulnaris. Needle one for the other. Needling under the ulnar tendon from the SI to the HT channel will usually resolve the condition, but it is sometimes necessary to needle into the tendon.

<u>Case Study:</u> Pg. 71, 124, 138, 141, 142, 143, 153.

Mu Guan, Gu Guan

<u>Indications:</u> Heel pain, plantar fasciitis.

<u>Location:</u> These points are located on either side of the center of the base of the palm.

<u>Needling information:</u> Needle perpendicularly, 0.5-1.0 cun in depth. Contralateral.

<u>Imaging:</u> Extremity image – palm of the hand is located at the plantar surface of the foot.

<u>Comments:</u> These Master Tong points are two needles at base of palm, near LU10, HT7.5. There is also a central point called Zong Guan. These are effective, but dissecting the anatomical correlates on the hand and foot show that using the pisiform as the calcaneus is clinically more effective. I will typically use 3-5 needles around the pisiform to treat heel pain. For arch of the foot, use an area just distal to PC7 – Zong Guan, and for the ball of the foot use the palmar side of the knuckles.

<u>Case Study:</u> Pg. 36, 135, 153

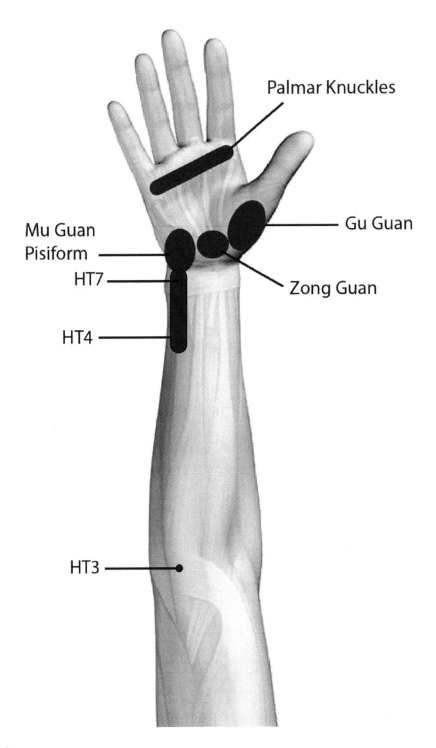

Palmar Knuckles

Gu Guan

Mu Guan
Pisiform

Zong Guan

HT7

HT4

HT3

Bodymapping Acupuncture Technique

SI3-5

Indications: Spinal pain in low back – GV channel. Sacrum pain – BL channel.

Location: This zone is located at the traditional location.

Needling information: Needle perpendicularly, 0.5-1.0 cun in depth. Contralateral.

Imaging: Torso image – wrist relates to L5-S1, hand relates to sacrum and coccyx.

Comments: This zone is used with Ling Gu, Da Bai, and SI Jt pt when needed.

Case Study: Pg. 24, 128, 130, 146, 152.

SI Joint Point

Indications:

1. Sacroiliac joint pain.

2. Deep ankle pain.

Location: Distal and medial to the styloid process of the ulna. Between SI6 and TW4.

Needling information: Needle perpendicularly, 0.5-1.5 cun in depth. Needle deeply into the pisoulnar ligament. Contralateral.

Imaging:

1. Torso image – wrist relates to L5-S1.

2. Extremity image – wrist relates to ankle.

Comments: This point is used with Ling Gu, Da Bai, and SI3,4, when needed. For the SI joint space, I find that needling into a joint works best and discovered this point distal and medial to the styloid process of the ulna. Needle from the SI channel deeply toward the HT channel through the pisoulnar ligament. This point only treats the joint space, not the muscles surrounding it. For the thoracolumbar fascia, use TW15 at the superior border of the scapula.

Case Study: Pg. 71, 130, 145, 147.

Gan Men

Indications: Rib pain, liver conditions, shingles, pancreatic symptoms.

Location: This area is located ½ way between elbow and wrist, above or below the ulna.

Needling information: Needle perpendicularly, 0.5-1.0 cun in depth. Contralateral.

Imaging: Torso image – forearm is located at the chest. SI is opposite clock with LR.

Comments: This Master Tung point can be needled above or below the ulna for different effects. The ulna is the border of the red and white skin, and therefore the border of yin and yang. I feel that yin treats organs and yang treats channels. Needle above the ulna in the yang area for channel pain along the ribs. Needle below the ulna on the left arm in the yin area for LR organ conditions. Needle below the ulna on the right arm for pancreatic conditions.

Case Study: Pg. 129, 131, 145, 150.

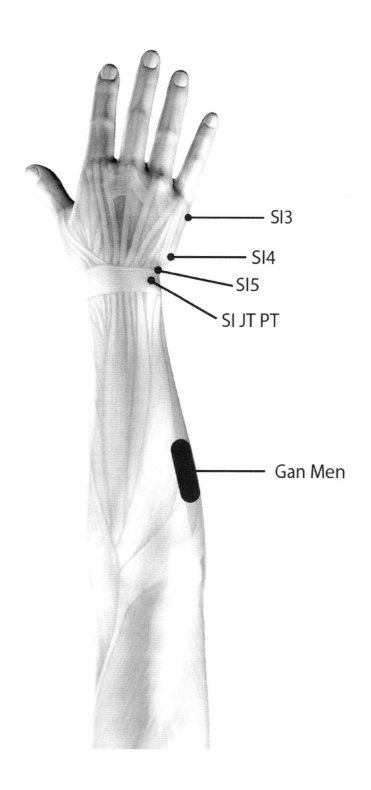

SI3

SI4

SI5

SI JT PT

Gan Men

Bodymapping Acupuncture Technique   95

SI9-10

Indications: Piriformis, obturator, gemellus and gluteus pain and tension.

Location: This zone is located at the traditional location, and encompasses an area from SI9-10 and all muscles in the area.

Needling information: Needle perpendicularly, 1.0-1.5 cun in depth. Contralateral.

Imaging: Extremity image – shoulder is located at the hip. SI is name pair with BL.

Comments: Needle any tender spots found in the infraspinatus, teres major and minor, 1-10 needles. The spine of the scapula relates to the iliac crest. Needle origins, insertions, and muscle bellies as needed.

Case Study: Pg. 37, 71, 130, 146, 148.

BL9-10

Indications: Heel pain at the calcaneus and Achilles attachment.

Location: This zone is located at the traditional location.

Needling information: Needle transversely, 0.5-1.0 cun in depth. Contralateral or ipsilateral.

Imaging: Torso image – the ankle is located at the neck.

Comments: Needle from BL9 toward BL10, 1-3 needles.

Case Study: Pg. 135, 153.

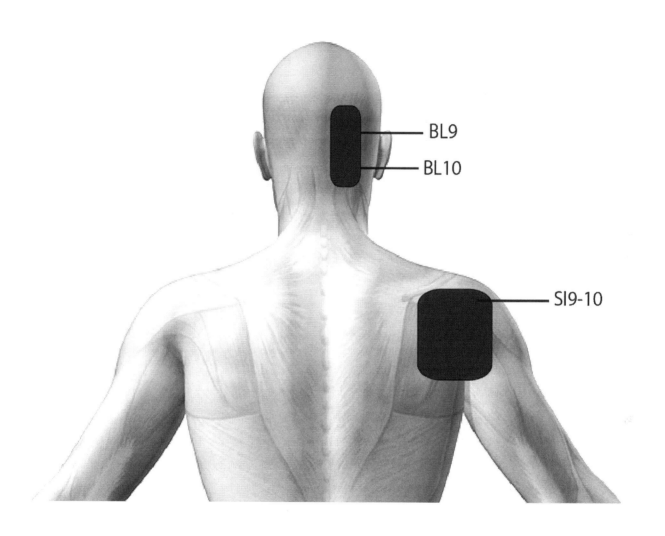

BL9

BL10

SI9-10

Bodymapping Acupuncture Technique   97

BL57 – Achilles tendon

Indications: Mid to upper back pain, BL channel.

Location: This zone is located from BL57 to the upper Achilles tendon.

Needling information: Needle perpendicularly, 0.5-1.5 cun in depth. Ipsilateral.

Imaging: Torso image – upper back is related to lower leg. BL treats itself.

Comments: The lumbar level is near BL40, needle from BL57 to the Achilles tendon for upper back pain. Very useful in combination with LU5-6.

Case Study: Pg. 127, 145.

BL58

Indications: BL channel quadratus lumborum muscle tension and pain, upper lumbar or lower thoracic pain, BL channel.

Location: This zone is located at the traditional location, and encompasses an area from BL58-40.

Needling information: Needle perpendicularly, 1.0-1.5 cun in depth. Ipsilateral.

Imaging: Torso image – knee is located at the navel. BL treats itself.

Comments: Use 1-3 needles to cover the area. Used in conjunction with LU5-6 zone and the Ling Gu set for spinal pain as well.

Case Study: Pg. 111, 114, 128, 130, 146.

Zheng Jin – Bo Qiu

Indications: Zheng Jin, Zheng Zong, Zheng Shi, Bo Qiu - pain along cervical spine, spinal fractures.

Location: On the Achilles tendon from the calcaneus to the gastrocnemius.

Needling information: Needle perpendicularly, 0.5-1.5 cun in depth. Can be needled to the back of the tibia. Contralateral or ipsilateral.

Imaging: Torso image – the ankle joint is located at the base of the skull. Tendon treats tendon, bone treats bone.

Comments: These are great Master Tung points (77.01-77.04) that are very effective at treating spinal pain on the cervical vertebra. Use two or more needles through Achilles tendon to tap on posterior tibia. The calcaneus is the occiput, and the place where the gastrocnemius muscle turns into tendon is the level of T1. Simply divide the tendon into 7 vertebra and needle where needed. It is only necessary to tap the tibia for relief in the most severe bone related conditions.

Case Study: Pg. 124, 125, 142.

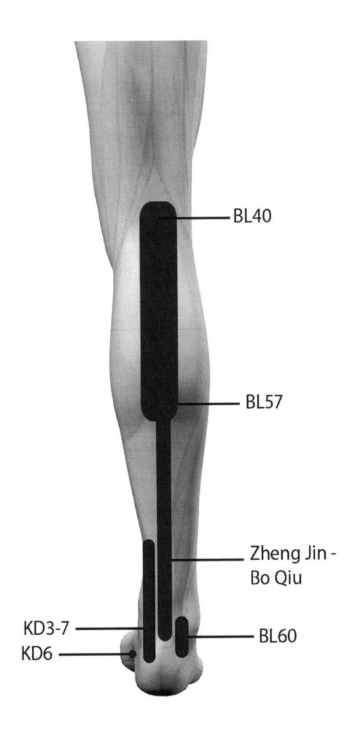

BL40

BL57

Zheng Jin -
Bo Qiu

KD3-7

KD6

BL60

BL60

Indications: Low back pain BL channel.

Location: This point is located at the traditional location.

Needling information: Needle transversely, 0.5-1.0 cun in depth. Ipsilateral.

Imaging: Torso image – ankle is located at L5-S1. BL treats itself.

Comments: Needle from the flat area of calcaneus near BL61 and thread into the hollow at BL60. Can also be needled into the junction of calcaneus and malleolus. Used in conjunction with the Ling Gu set for spinal pain as well.

Case Study: Pg. 37, 71, 128, 130, 146.

KD3-7

Indications:

1. Sternocleidomastoid muscle pain, scalene muscle pain at the LI channel, thoracic outlet syndrome at the LI channel.

2. Tonsillitis, swollen lymph under jaw.

3. Low back pain.

Location:

1. This zone is located at the traditional area from KD3-7.

2. This zone is located at the traditional area from KD5-3

3. This point is located from the flat of the medial calcaneus toward KD5,4,3.

<u>Needling information:</u> 0.5-1.0 cun in depth.

1. Needle from the traditional location of KD3 to KD7, close to the Achilles tendon. Contralateral.

2. Needle obliquely from the traditional location of KD5 toward KD4 and KD3. Contralateral.

3. Needle obliquely from the flat of the calcaneus through the traditional location of KD5 toward the hollow of KD4 and KD3. Can also be needled into the junction of calcaneus and malleolus. Contralateral or ipsilateral.

<u>Imaging:</u>

1-2. Torso image – the ankle joint is located at the base of the skull. KD is opposite clock with LI.

3. Torso image – the ankle is located at the L5-S1 area. KD is yin yang pair with BL, KD treats itself.

<u>Comments:</u>

1-2. KD5 is at the tonsil and lymph level under the jaw, KD3 is at the muscle origins of the scalene, and KD7 is at the clavicle, 1st rib, and LI16 medial to the acromion process. Use 1-3 needles from KD3-7 for thoracic outlet syndrome and LI channel scalene pain. Occasionally pain palpated at GB21 is not relieved with HT4 and this zone works well to treat the LI channel underneath.

3. KD pairs with BL and with itself to treat the low back. By needling from the calcaneus into the hollow of KD3, the joint space is crossed and it treats the spinal joints better.

<u>Case Study:</u> Pg. 71, 113, 125, 138, 139, 141, 143, 144, 146.

KD6

Indications: Hara zone: kidney area below the navel, menstrual cramps.

Location: This point is located between KD2 and KD6, below the junction of the talus and navicular bones into the deep recess of the arch.

Needling information: Needle perpendicularly, 0.5-1.2 cun in depth.

Imaging: Extended extremity image – the foot is located at the base of the torso. KD treats itself. Either side or bilateral.

Comments: For hara release of kidney zone: needle deeply either side or bilateral for menstrual cramps or lower central abdominal pain.

Case Study: Pg. 134.

KD22-27

Indications:

1. Rib pain at the BL channel in the mid and upper back.

2. Pubic tubercle and symphysis pain.

3. Inguinal ligament pain.

Location: This zone is located at the classical location of these points. KD27 extends from the jugular notch of the manubrium to the medial border of the coracoid process.

Needling information:

1. Needle obliquely, 0.5-1.0 cun in depth. Thread the needle medial or lateral, being careful of the lungs. Ipsilateral.

2. Needle KD27 at the junction of the clavicle and manubrium.

3. Needle KD27 toward LU2 and the coracoid process, angling between the 1st rib and the clavicle.

Imaging:

1. Torso image – chest relates front to back.

2-3. Torso image – chest relates top to bottom.

Comments:

1. These are very good at treating rib pain near the spine. Look for tender spots at the junction of the rib at the sternum, or between the ribs in the intercostal spaces. Needle the front for the back at the same level. 1-5 needles.

2. Needle closer to the jugular notch of the manubrium to treat the pubic symphysis and the muscle attachments there.

3. Needling along the subclavius muscle to treat inguinal ligament is a great way to release tension in the groin area. I think that ligaments can have tension just like muscles and can be treated similarly.

Case Study: Pg. 71, 127, 144, 148.

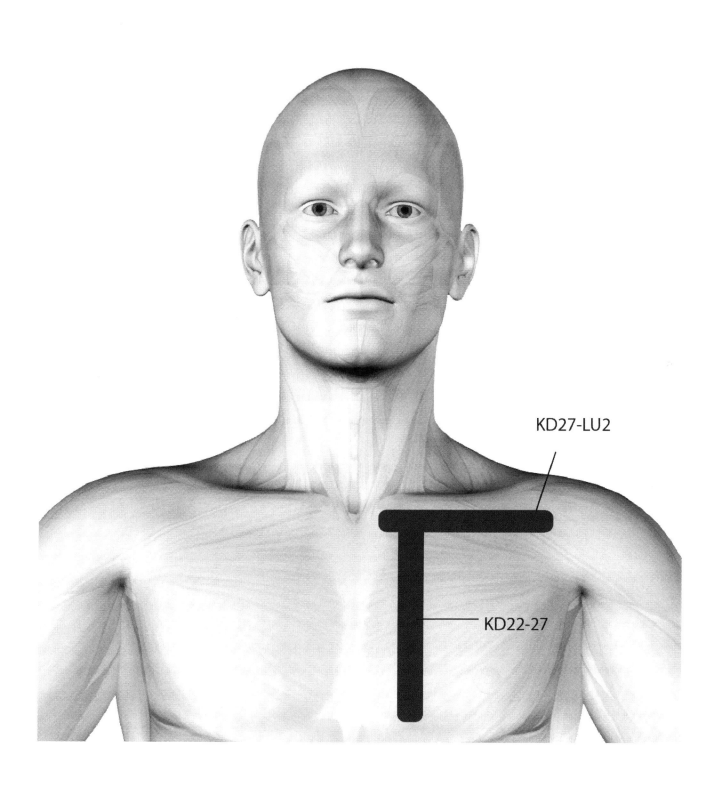

KD27-LU2

KD22-27

PC3.5

Indications: Deep sinus pain or stagnation at ST1-3.

Location: This point is located between PC3 and PC4.

Needling information: Needle perpendicularly, 0.5-1.5 cun in depth. Contralateral.

Imaging: Head image – the nose is located just below the elbow. PC is opposite clock with ST.

Comments: There are many good points for sinus pain like LI4, SP9 and ST36. This point can treat the deepest areas of the sinuses and can be needled deeply.

PC4

Indications: ST5-6 muscle tension or pain at the masseter muscle.

Location: This point is located at the traditional location.

Needling information: Needle perpendicularly, 0.5-1.0 cun in depth. Contralateral.

Imaging: Head image – mouth is located at mid forearm. PC is opposite clock with ST.

Comments: The mouth is open in the image. PC4 is located at the midpoint of the mouth, needling a little above or below will treat the upper or lower jaw respectively.

Case Study: Pg. 122, 140.

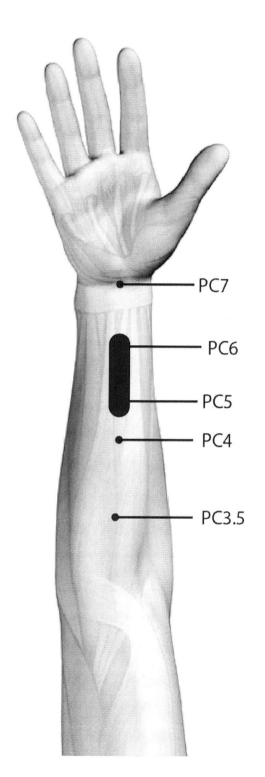

PC7

PC6

PC5

PC4

PC3.5

Bodymapping Acupuncture Technique

PC5-6

Indications:

1. ST channel tooth pain.

2. Tongue pain or lack of taste, difficulty swallowing.

3. Chest or breast pain ST channel.

4. Hara zones: stomach or heart area.

5. Knee pain and swelling.

Location: This zone is located at the traditional location.

Needling information: Needle perpendicularly, 0.5-1.0 cun in depth. Contralateral.

Imaging: PC is opposite clock with ST. PC treats itself.

1-2. Head image – mouth is located at mid forearm.

3-4. Torso image – chest is located at the forearm.

Comments:

1. The mouth is open in the image. The lower jaw is ST channel and PC5 is located at the lower jaw, lower teeth, and tonguc.

2. The tongue is involved with many aspects of eating and descending food to the stomach; taste, the movement of food around the mouth, and the swallowing function. The tongue is also a muscle and therefor earth. For these reasons I believe the tongue is ST channel, treat it with opposite clock PC.

3. The chest is KD, ST and PC channels. This point treats both ST and itself PC.

4. For hara release of stomach or heart zones: ST area - PC6 either side or bilateral, HT area - PC6 either side or bilateral.

5. For knee pain, especially when there is swelling, needle contralateral. Use with deep LR3 ipsilateral. This is a Master Tung treatment for knee pain. I believe this point works by increasing the blood flow through the knee joint, and seems to work best when there

Bodymapping Acupuncture Technique

is swelling and tightness around the knee. The combination with LR3 on the same side of the knee pain activates the blood flow by needling near deep arteries. I will typically not place any other needles on the affected leg, and have the patient "pump" the knee ten times every ten minutes. The swelling will usually resolve during the treatment, and range of motion will increase.

Case Study: Pg. 79, 83, 125, 132, 134, 138, 140, 147, 149, 154.

PC7

Indications:

1. ST9-12 area pain.

2. Sore throat on the ST channel.

Location: This point is located in the classical location.

Needling information: Needle perpendicularly, or oblique distally, 0.5-1.0 cun in depth. Contralateral.

Imaging: Torso image – the base of the neck is located at the wrist. PC is opposite clock with ST.

Comments: This point is needled from PC6 toward PC7 depending on the level of condition. The wrist crease is the base of the chin and top of the throat. The closer to PC6, the further down the neck the point treats. If the condition is central and on the CV channel, needle both sides. Very rare CV channel cases will need the GV needled on the cervicals to treat the condition.

Case Study: Pg. 125, 141, 153.

TW15

Indications: Gluteus maximus attachment at the thoracolumbar fascia and sacrum.

Location: This point is located at the traditional location.

Needling information: Needle perpendicularly, 0.5-1.0 cun in depth. Contralateral.

Imaging: Extremity image – shoulder is located at the hip.

Comments: This point treats the soft tissue around the SI joint, use the SI Jt Pt for deeper joint pain and tightness.

Case Study: Pg. 94, 129, 131, 147.

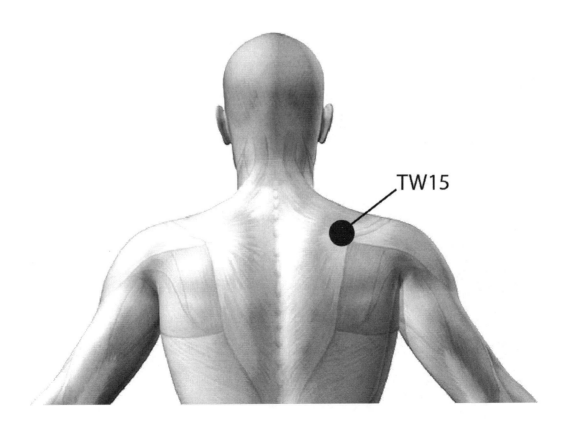

GB32-34

Indications:

1. Temporal muscle pain at GB channel, temporomandibular joint pain.

2. Rib pain on GB channel.

Location: These points are located in a zone between the traditional locations.

Needling information: Needle perpendicularly, 1.0-1.5 cun in depth. Ipsilateral.

Imaging:

1. Head image – jaw is located at the knee joint, and the temporal lobe at distal thigh. The tendinous nature of this point location helps treat tight muscle attachments and joint spaces. GB treats itself distally.

2. Torso image – knee is located at navel.

Comments:

1. These points are very effective at releasing a tight jaw and a narrow mouth opening. They are also good for a popping sound when the mouth is opened. Look for tender points along the distal iliotibial tract to its insertion at the fibular head.

2. GB33-34 treats rib pain on GB channel. It treats 12th rib when combined with BL58 and Gan Men yang area.

Case Study: Pg. 122, 129, 132, 138, 141, 145.

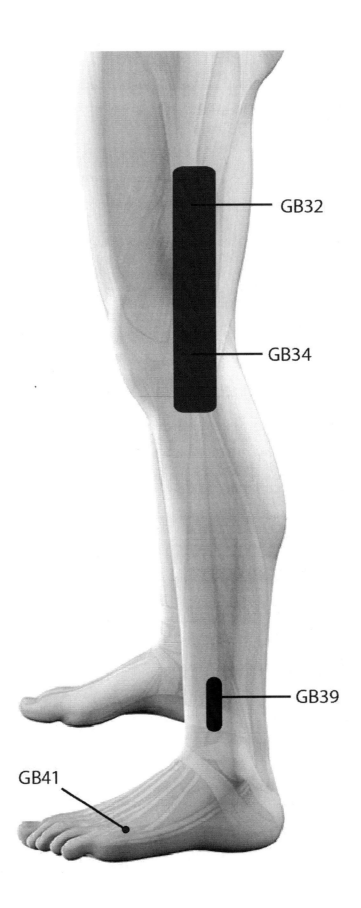

GB32

GB34

GB39

GB41

GB39

Indications: Subscapularis muscle pain.

Location: This point is located at the level of GB39. 3cun superior to the lateral malleolus, between the fibula and tibia, and on the medial side of the fibula.

Needling information: Needle perpendicularly, 0.5-1.5 cun in depth. Contralateral.

Imaging: Torso image – the neck is located at the ankle, upper back at the lower leg. GB is opposite clock with HT.

Comments: In searching for a way to treat subscapularis pain, KD3 had some effect on a patient. This got me thinking about how and why which led to the conclusion that subscapularis is HT channel. Opposite clock is GB, and after trying a number of GB points in the area of the upper back, this frontal GB39 seems to work best. It should be needled deeply to the interosseus membrane because the muscle is deep. 1-2 needles.

Case Study: Pg. 71, 126, 141, 143, 144.

GB41

Indications: Belt channel pain along QL and psoas/iliacus.

Location: This point is located at the traditional location.

Needling information: Needle distally under the extensor tendon toward GB42, 0.5-1.0 cun in depth. Ipsilateral.

Imaging: Extended extremity image – ankle is located at hip, foot extends onto pelvis. GB treats itself.

Comments: Quadratus lumborum is BL and belt channel. Treat BL with BL58 zone, belt channel with GB41. Psoas is released with pec minor, but it can also be belt channel stagnation and released with GB41. Iliacus is related with subscapularis, but being hard to needle, GB41 works well.

Case Study: Pg. 71, 129, 130, 139, 145, 150.

LR3.5

Indications: SI18 area pain for the teeth, gums, or face.

Location: This point is located on a flat area on the medial cuneiform, between LR3 and LR4.

Needling information: Needle transversely, 0.5-.75 cun in depth. Contralateral. Thread under the extensor hallucis longus tendon.

Imaging: Torso image – nose and zygomatic arch are located at mid foot. LR is opposite clock with SI.

Comments: This point was discovered while looking for a way to treat pain under the zygomatic arch for trigeminal neuralgia. It is also useful for maxilla and tooth pain in the same area.

Case Study: Pg. 71, 137.

LR5

Indications: Rhomboid pain, upper back pain.

Location: This point is a zone that extends from the traditional location of LR5 distal toward LR4.

Needling information: Needle obliquely, 0.5-1.0 cun in depth. Thread across the tibia, from the proximal front ridge near ST channel to the distal medial border toward SP channel. Contralateral.

Imaging: Torso image – the neck is located at the ankle, upper back at the lower leg. LR is opposite clock with SI.

Comments: This zone will treat the rhomboid muscle. Needle proximally for the lower rhomboid and distally for the upper.

Case Study: Pg. 126, 138, 141, 143, 143.

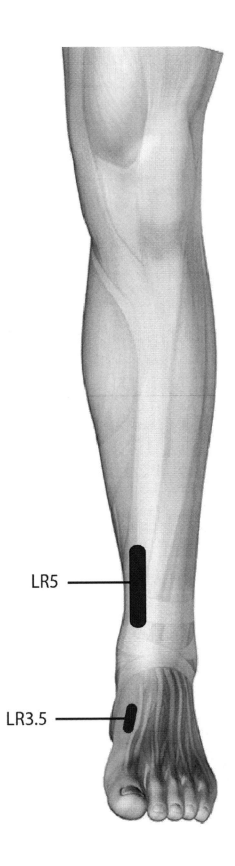

LR5

LR3.5

CV9-15

Indications: GV pain in mid to lower back.

Location: This zone is located at the classical location of these points.

Needling information: Needle perpendicularly, 0.5-1.0 cun in depth.

Imaging: Torso image – torso relates front to back.

Comments: When spinal pain continues after treating all the muscles around it, needle the front for the back at the same level.

Case Study: Pg. 127.

CV15-22

Indications: GV pain in mid and upper back.

Location: This zone is located at the classical location of these points.

Needling information: Needle transversely, 0.5-1.0 cun in depth. Thread the needle proximal or distal.

Imaging: Torso image – chest relates front to back.

Comments: When spinal pain continues after treating all the muscles around it, needle the front for the back at the same level.

Case Study: Pg. 127, 144.

CV22-24

Indications: GV14-16 pain.

Location: This zone is located at the classical location of these points.

Needling information: Needle transversely, 0.5-1.0 cun in depth. Thread the needle proximal or distal.

Imaging: Torso image – chest relates front to back.

Comments: When spinal pain continues after treating all the muscles around it, needle the front for the back at the same level.

Case Study: Pg. 38, 124, 144.

GV20

Indications: Coccyx pain, hemorrhoids.

Location: This point is located at the traditional location.

Needling information: Needle obliquely, 0.5-1.0 cun in depth.

Imaging: Torso image – top treats bottom.

Comments: Needle anterior to posterior from GV20 back, angling the needles to create a wedge shape (2 needles).

Case Study: Pg. 131, 139, 147, 149, 153.

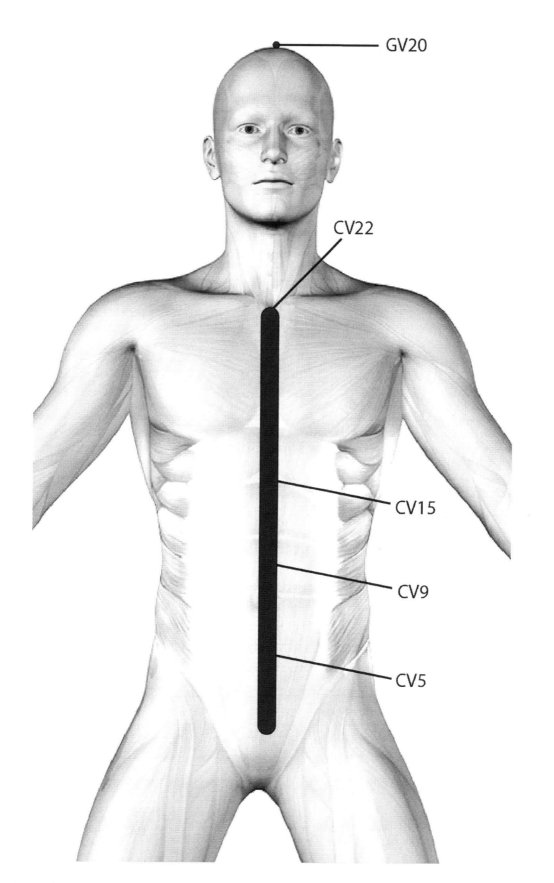

GV20

CV22

CV15

CV9

CV5

Bodymapping Acupuncture Technique

119

Chapter 2: Strategies and Favorite Points by Diseased Location

Where is it now?

Diagnosing channel pain

When using distal point acupuncture, results are often immediate. This is wonderful and proves to the patient and ourselves the effectiveness of acupuncture, our points, and our profession. Because the effects are so quick, pain and symptoms will seem to move around as we are needling. This may not be wind as we are often taught, but the un-layering of a condition.

Most patients that come into the clinic have had their symptoms for a period of time. This leads to compensation around the effected area and corresponding areas.

As we are needling and pain is lessening, it is important to ask the patient a simple question. Where is it now? The answer will confirm that we have treated all effected channels and anatomy, or that there are more layers to treat. Continue conjugating the channels and images until all layers are resolved. This can take many needles at times, and we need to be mindful of the tolerances of the patient. These layers mostly resolve in order of their appearance. The condition will tend to centralize, or to reverse in that order and become focussed on the one spot that was the original injury. This can happen in one treatment, or take many.

Head

We find the most effective image for treating the head is either the hand and foot correlation, or the whole head on the arm or leg. Think of the areas around the knee and elbow as an expanded eye level, a little above or below the joint will still have effect on eye level. The ears are at both the eye level and the neck level and will often need needles in both image locations. We find that treating the channel that travels around the ear (TW) most effective for the treatment of ear conditions. The TMJ problems have 2 channels involved, GB and ST. SI and ST channels both have internal paths that manifest superficially further along their channels (SI18, ST8). We find the tongue is ST channel rather than the usual HT.

Headache

Headaches are usually on multiple channels and need multiple points to treat. For frontal headache that travels across the forehead, we would start with HT3 and LU5 bilateral. If at the temples, needle SP9 opposite side, if still at the front, and more of a severe pain, needle HT8, LU10. These last two points are used for the very worst cases, and many patients prefer the less painful points at the elbow. ST channel is not included as it is not seen clinically as often as the others. It can be treated with same channel (ST36 same side), name pair (LI4 same or opposite side), or clock opposite (PC3 opposite side).

These points are all either head reflected on arm or leg image, or torso reflected on arm or leg image and using the clock opposite channel relationship.

HT8, LU10 are also used for the very worst cases, but many patients prefer the less painful points at the elbow. ST channel is not included as it is not seen clinically as often as the others. It can be treated with same channel (ST36 ipsilateral), name pair (LI4 ipsilateral or contralateral), or clock opposite (PC3 contralateral).

HT 03: GB channel headache at eye level, eye pain at GB1.

LU 05: BL channel headache at eye level, eye pain at BL1-2. (can also help if the headache is on or close to the GV channel).

SP 09: TW channel headache, temple headache, ear problems.

HT 07: Vertex headache on GB channel, occipital headache on GB channel (needle from lateral side under ulnar tendon).

LU 09: Vertex headache on BL channel, occipital headache on BL channel (can be useful for GV also, try to thread along channel distally, occasionally LU9-10 is useful if the pain radiates onto the occiput).

TMD

HT3: GB2 pain, joint popping or temporalis muscle pain.

PC4: ST5-6 muscle tension or pain at the masseter muscle.

GB32-34: Temporal muscle pain at GB channel, temporomandibular joint pain.

Neck

The neck is complex with many crossing channels. Most patients with neck conditions will get more needles than other areas of the body. We find that treating all channels near the ones specifically involved is a good practice as many muscle layers can hide the involvement of other channels. Cervical pain is either the muscle attachments and the nuchal tendon, or the spinous processes themselves. We usually start by treating the muscles, and after they are relaxed, check the cervical again. If the pain is still there, not only is the condition more advanced, it will require treating the tendon and spinous process as well with upright tendon, or CV points.

Diagnosing Thoracic Outlet Syndrome

When a patient presents with numb, tingling and/or pain in the fingers or hand, what are the best strategies? Lets start with the diagnosis. Many patients will have been diagnosed with carpal tunnel syndrome. This is one possible cause, very well treated with contralateral LR5-7 zone, but I often find the neck muscles involved. Palpate the neck muscles and cervical spine. If there is no cervical spinal pain, and all the pain is muscle related, then the most common condition is thoracic outlet syndrome.

The brachial plexus nerve bundle as well as vascular tissue pass next to and sometimes through (a variance in anatomy) the scalene muscles. The scalene muscles originate at the vertebra, and insert on the 1st or 2nd ribs. If these muscles are tight, the brachial plexus and blood flow can be restricted to the arms, causing numb and tingly sensations.

Different points are treated depending on which fingers or parts of the hand are effected. If you place the hand on the shoulder thumb forward the channels line up like this:

> The thumb with the LU channel
> The 2nd finger with the LI channel
> The 3rd finger with the GB channel
> The 4th finger with the TW channel
> The 5th finger with the SI channel.

Treat the finger involved with the channel associated with it. For LU and the upper chest under the clavicle, use SP5/LR4. For the LI and scalene muscles, use KD3-7. For the GB and trapezius muscles, use HT4-6. For the TW and levator scapula, use SP5.5. For the SI and scapula or rhomboid, use LR5. All points are contralateral, and needled with multiple points in the zone.

Usually more than one finger or area is involved, and multiple points need to be needled. The symptoms could of course be coming from the brain, cervical vertebra, or arm, and those would require further diagnostics and treatments. This strategy is useful when the symptoms are caused by muscle tightness and tension.

Neck Pain

Neck palpation and treatment

Palpation is important here. If the pain is on the spine with or without muscle tightness and tenderness, needle the LU7-9 zone at the appropriate level. If the muscle tension is relieved, check the spine. If the spine is better, it was the tight muscles pulling on the attachments, if the spine is still tender, the condition is deeper. It could be the nuchal ligament, treated well with the Achilles tendon points, Zheng Jin – Zheng Shi. It could also be a disk problem or stenosis, a narrowing of the bony canal the nerve passes through. Depending on the reason for the disk problem, relaxing the muscles and increasing circulation will help, but postural exercises are necessary to correct the curvature and push the disk back into position. The McKenzie Method is a favorite. Once in position it will heal that way. This can take many months for a curative state. If the problem is stenosis, I believe that it may eventually need surgery to remove bone that is compressing the nerve. Acupuncture can provide some temporary relief. Many times even if medical imaging shows stenosis, there may be many factors contributing to the condition. The muscle tightness and disk bulging are treatable, and removing just one of the factors can give long term relief.

CV22-24: GV14-16 pain.

PC7: ST9-12 area pain.

LU7-9: BL channel neck pain and conditions BL10-11 area, base of skull to T1 level.

HT4-7: GB channel neck pain and conditions from the base of skull to T1 level (needle from lateral side of ulnar tendon).

SP5/LR4: SI17 or TW16-17 area pain at corner of jaw, scalene muscle pain at the TW or

SI channels. Ear pain and problems at the neck level, ear infection.

KD3-7: Sternocleidomastoid muscle pain, scalene muscle pain at the LI channel, thoracic outlet syndrome at the LI channel.

Zheng Jin-Bo Qiu: Zheng Jin, Zheng Zong, Zheng Shi, Bo Qiu - pain along cervical spine, spinal fractures (two or more needles through Achilles tendon to tap on posterior tibia).

Throat conditions

The throat is CV, ST, and LI. LI5 is a great point to treat both ST and LI at the throat. There is a hollow at the "anatomical snuffbox", needle from the distal or proximal side into the hollow. KD3 is also very useful for swollen lymph and tonsillitis. Look for tender and "gummy" areas.

LI5: Sore throat of any kind.

PC7: Sore throat on the ST channel.

PC5: Tongue pain or lack of taste, difficulty swallowing.

KD3-7: Tonsillitis, swollen lymph under jaw.

Back

The back includes upper back, mid back and lower back. All have BL, KD, and GV channels. Upper back also has TW, SI, HT, and some LI under the trapezius at GB21.

Mid and upper back have ribs which include GB, LR (mostly on lower mid back ribs), and internally SP.

Low back pain is mostly BL with some KD and GV involved on the spine. LU, BL, and SI are used to treat the BL channel. LI, KD, and BL are used to treat the KD channel. CV is used to treat GV. The low back also has the belt channel traveling through it, which ties together L2-5, paraspinal muscles, quadratus lumborum, oblique, ASIS, psoas, iliacus, and the reproductive organs (especially female).

Upper back pain

Chong Zi – Chong Xian: Rhomboid pain, upper back pain, works best if there is a history of lung issues (two needles near LU10, look for veins).

SP5.5: Levator scapula muscle insertion pain at the superior angle of the scapula (low SP6).

LR5: Rhomboid pain, upper back pain (thread across tibia).

GB39: Subscapularis muscle pain (treats HT channel, needle into interosseus membrane).

CV15-22: GV pain in mid and upper back.

KD22-27: Rib pain at the BL channel in the mid and upper back.

Mid back pain

LU5-6: BL channel quadratus lumborum muscle tension and pain, upper lumbar or lower thoracic pain, BL channel.

HT3: Lower rib and flank pain. Herpes zoster or shingles on GB channel.

CV9-15: GV pain in mid to lower back.

BL57-Achilles tendon: Mid to upper back pain, BL channel.

Low back pain

Low back palpation and treatment

For low back pain anywhere palpation is very important for diagnosis of muscle and channel stagnation. I usually have patients lying supine, with pillows under their head and knees, and run my hand between their back and the table. The patients typically do not need to de-clothe, and are requested to wear loose comfortable clothing. With them lying in this position, the muscles are usually in their most relaxed state. Some patients are in too much pain to lay in this position, and we have recliners available for them, though it is more difficult to palpate this way.

When palpating some patients will state that the pain is not where you are pressing, but they often will have tight and tender areas that are involved in other areas than where they feel the condition. I tell them that I am going to palpate all around and we will see what we find. I start by palpating from the R or L side of the table. I check the spine from L5 up to T10 looking at their face for signs of pain or discomfort. I am also feeling for whether the spine is slightly moveable or not, and at what level. I check along the paraspinal muscles next to the spine, and pay special attention to L5-S1 and the sacroiliac joint.

I then check the area around and just below the SI joint; the gluteus maximus, minimus deeply, medius, and lower the piriformis. There is also obturator and gemellus attachments near the coccyx. I check the ischial tuberosity at the attachment of the hamstrings, and on the lateral side at the attachment of quadratus femoris. Then I palpate the attachments at the trochanter. If any of these muscles are tender, I will start at the origin or insertion and palpate the length of the tissue. Travel down gluteus maximus and palpate the iliotibial tract for tenderness. Most patients will have IT pain, but it may not be adding to their condition.

Many patients will think they have piriformis pain, but it may end up being gluteus or obturator, and this thorough examination will help to determine the worst areas. The reason for all this palpation is that each area involved has different points to treat it. Piriformis is best treated with teres minor in the opposing shoulder, but gluteus pain at the iliac crest is best treated with infraspinatus along the spine of the scapula.

I then go back up to quadratus lumborum and check around the paraspinals, under and at the 12th rib, and travel outward toward the GB channel at the obliques. Traveling along the belt channel, palpate over the iliac crest and down to the anterior superior iliac spine. Palpate just medial to the ASIS with gentle pressure increasing to tolerance to feel the psoas and along the iliac fossa the iliacus. These are important areas because they can pull on the lumbar spine, causing back pain, and they have varying treatments, so it is good to differentiate if possible. At the ASIS palpate medial and slightly distal to check the inguinal ligament for tenderness. If the patient is not complaining of pain at the pubic bone, I typically will not palpate down the inguinal ligament to the attachment at the pubic tubercle, as this can be uncomfortable. From the ASIS palpate laterally the tensor fascia lata.

Spinal pain any level: Ling Gu, Da Bai, SI3,4,5(1-3 needles), BL58 (ipsilateral, 1-3 needles), BL60, CV4-7 (2-5 needles).

Paraspinal pain: add LU5-6 (1-3 needles).

QL pain: add GB41 ipsilateral.

SI joint pain: SI joint point.

Thoracolumbar fascia around SI joint: TW15.

12th rib: LU5-6, BL58(ipsilateral), Gan Men, GB34(ipsilateral, 1-3 needles), GB41.

Gluteus muscles: infraspinatus along the spine of the scapula and the belly of the muscle, posterior and lateral deltoid.

Piriformis, obturator, gemellus: teres minor(needle origin, belly or insertion as needed).

IT: lateral deltoid traveling down the TW channel(1-10 needles).

ASIS: coracoid process.

Inguinal ligament: subclavius(1-3 needles carefully oblique between the clavicle and the 1st rib).

TFL: short head of biceps and coracobrachialis

Psoas: GB41 ipsilateral, pec minor.

Iliacus: GB41 ipsilateral

12th Rib Pain

12th rib pain is a tender spot palpated from the oblique into the edge of the 12th rib. It is the overlapping of 3 channels: BL, GB, and LR (I think all lower ribs have both LR and GB). It usually requires LU5-6 and Gan Men contralateral, GB34 and BL58 ipsilateral. If QL is also involved, GB41 same side is helpful as well.

All low back points

Ling Gu: Low back pain and sciatica (proximal to LI4, just distal to the junction of the first two metacarpals).

Da Bai: Low back pain and sciatica, assistant to Ling Gu, located at LI3.

SI3-5: Spinal pain in low back – GV channel. Sacrum pain – BL channel. Works well with Ling Gu, Da Bai.

SI joint point: Sacroiliac joint pain. Needle deeply slightly distal and medial to the styloid process of the ulna into the pisoulnar ligament.

BL58: BL channel quadratus lumborum muscle tension and pain, upper lumbar or lower thoracic paraspinal pain, BL channel. 1-3 needles, zone from BL58-40.

BL60: Low back pain (needle from BL61 to 60, or into junction of calcaneous and malleolus).

KD5-3: Low back pain (needle from KD5–3, or into junction of calcaneous and malleolus).

GB41: Belt channel pain along QL and psoas/iliacus (needle distally under extensor tendon).

SI9-10: Piriformis, obturator, gemellus and gluteus pain and tension (needle any tender spots found in the infraspinatus, teres major and minor, 1-10 needles).

TW15: Gluteus maximus attachment at the thoracolumbar fascia and sacrum.(this point treats the tender soft tissue around the SI joint, use the SI jt pt for deeper joint pain and tightness).

GV20: Coccyx pain, hemorrhoids (needle anterior to posterior from GV20, angling the needles to create a wedge shape).

Frontal Torso

Chest

LI6-8: Chest pain on KD or ST channels (thread needle along LI channel).

Gan Men: Rib pain, liver conditions, shingles, pancreatic symptoms (½ way between elbow and wrist, yang above or yin below ulna).

Shingles

If on the ribs, in the most common hypochondriac location, channels involved are LR, GB, BL. Use LU5-6, HT3-4, Gan Men yang area. See case study Pg. 149.

PC5-6: Chest or breast pain ST channel.

GB33-34: Rib pain on GB channel.

ST32: Chest pain, physical heart problems (2 needles 1.5 cun).

ST38-39: Breast pain on sides of breasts, breast lumps, breast fibroids, breast tenderness with menstruation (needle from ST38-41).

SP5/LR4: LU1-2 area pain.

LU1-2: Pain and tenderness at the ASIS (anterior superior iliac spine), TFL (tensor fascia lata) pain or tenderness, psoas pain.

Hara Diagnosis and Abdominal Pain

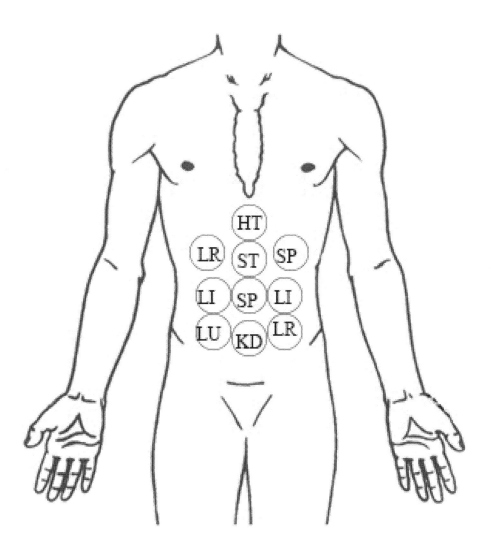

    This style of hara diagnosis comes from the Nanjing. There are similarities with other styles of acupuncture, especially Japanese techniques. There are specific zones with release points. These are very useful in helping diagnose internal organ problems, and also in treating abdominal problems. If nothing else they can help with an understanding of deeper imbalances. The points should have immediate effect, and pain or discomfort should resolve almost instantly. These palpation areas are useful for diagnostic purposes as well as treatment areas for abdominal symptoms. Palpate the areas looking for tightness or tenderness. Areas should release immediately after needling the appropriate point.

HT area: PC6, either side or bilateral.

LR area upper R quadrant: LR4 same side.

ST area: PC6, either side or bilateral.

SP area upper L quadrant: SP9 same side (this is often seen with pancreatic problems).

LI area R of the navel: ST36-37 same side (may take 2 needles).

SP area central: SP9, either side or bilateral.

LI area L of the navel: ST36-37 same side (may take 2 needles).

LU area lower R quadrant: LI10 opposite side (may take 2 needles).

KD area: KD6, either side or bilateral (abdominal menstrual cramps are often located here and resolve immediately with this point).

LR area lower L quadrant: LR4 same side.

Extremities and Other

PC6: Knee pain, swelling, and circulation (contralateral, use with deep LR3 ipsilateral).

Mu Guan, Gu Guan: Heel pain, plantar fasciitis (two needles on either side of the center of the base of the palm. The anatomical location of these points using the pisiform as the calcaneus is clinically more effective).

BL9-10: Heel pain at the calcaneus and Achilles attachment. Needle from BL9 toward BL10.

Section V: Case Studies, Examples and Explanations

Head

Trigeminal neuralgia

"The Carol Slider"

Middle aged Caucasian woman came in presenting with trigeminal neuralgia on the L side for 6yrs. Pain was a 8-10/10 constant, depending on the time of day and exertion. She was taking multiple pain medications. Channels involved: GB, BL, TW, ST, LI. In an earlier version of the channel chart, I did not have SI18 represented. The reason was that I made the patients results prove the channel locations through multiple treatments. It took over 5 years, more than 30,000 patient visits, and 20+ revisions to get the chart the way it is now. I am sure it is still not exact, but close. At least for the superficial tissues.

GB has the largest area involved, so we started with right side HT8,3. That helped about 50%. We added right - LU10,5, ST36,37, LI4,3 and left – LI4,3, ST36,37. We repeated these treatments 2x per week for 1 month with little variation in the points.

At this point the pain was much less, but there was one spot we just could not get to go away. It was just under the zygomatic arch on the Left side. We tried many variations of ST and LI points, images, and relationships. Nothing changed it. I finally went over to the channel chart on the wall and saw SI18 staring back at me. I had not had one patient in all that time with pain on SI18 that did not go away with ST and LI treatments, so I left SI18 off the chart. I went through the conjugation. Torso image, use clock opposite SI – LR, and the level on the foot would be..... right where there is no point! Somewhere between LR3-4, LR3.5. We palpated around and found a very tender spot on a flat surface on the medial cuneiform and navicular, under the extensor hallucis longus. Needle transverse and medial toward lateral under the tendon. She felt the relief before I even asked her.... "oh, that's it! You got it!" It only took a few more treatments to get complete relief. We added SI18 to the chart. If you notice there is no connecting channel on the chart from SI17 to SI18. It is internal. We have treated many patients with maxilla pain, and many are SI related, especially when the upper teeth are involved.

Since Carol was an avid baseball fan, and this point slides under the tendon, we named it "The Carol Slider".

Vertex headache

"Shari"

Shari presented with vertex headache. She was a 34 Yr old woman and had the headache for 3 days. The pain was on the BL, GB, and GV channels. We needled LU9 and HT7 both bilaterally. The pain resolved immediately and she said it felt like someone was unzipping the headache off her head. She also had some nausea and neck tension. We needled PC6, HT4, LU7, SP5/LR4, SP5.5, LR5, and KD3-7. Some of the neck pain was in the lateral scalene muscle on LI, TW and SI channels.

Easy jaw pain

"Tess"

43 Yr old woman came in with jaw pain after a long weekend of family gathering. She was not sure whether it was stress from the family or the continuous eating and talking that caused her pain. She could only open her mouth 1-2 fingers. I needled GB32-34 with 3 needles bilaterally, and she could open her mouth 2-3 fingers. I added HT3 bilateral and over the course of the treatment she got open to 3 fingers. After 2 treatments the condition was resolved.

"I can't taste anything!"

"Beth"

67 Yr old woman presented with lack of taste after chemotherapy. She had two rounds of chemotherapy and radiation for throat cancer, and had lost her taste completely 6 months previous. The cancer was in remission, but her taste had not come

back. Her medical professionals had told her at this point it probably would not return.

We started with treating the classical tongue channel the HT. Opposite clock GB mouth level did not seem to help after 3 treatments. We used GB41, GB38, LI4, and GV20.

I started to think what channel would logically go to the tongue? Taste is associated with the digestion, as is swallowing. The tongue is also a muscle, and therefor earth. The first digestive organ food goes to is the stomach.

Opposite clock ST is PC, mouth level is around PC5. After 2 treatments with PC5 bilateral, ST 36 and 40 bilateral, LI4 bilateral, and LR3 bilateral, her taste started coming back. After another 5 treatments she was happy with the results even though there was not a complete recovery.

Infectious vertigo

"Jody"

67 Yr old woman presented with right sided inner ear infection and vertigo. She had a hard time coming into the clinic because of the strong nausea she was experiencing. She was more comfortable resting in a recliner than on a table. The ear is at a meeting of two images. Because of the largeness of the face in comparison to the rest of the head, the ear falls at both eye level and base of skull. Two points are needed to treat the entire ear. The channel that travels around the ear is TW, and opposite clock is SP.

I needled SP9 with 2 needles bilateral, and SP5/LR4 with 3 needles on the left and 2 on the right. Knee is eye level and ankle is base of skull level. This relieved 60% of the pain. I then added KD3-7 x2, and PC6 bilateral. The nausea reduced and the vertigo eased a little. By the end of the treatment, her pain was 75% better and she could get up with much less difficulty. Two days later she came back for a follow up treatment, still 50% better. After the above points again, the pain was 80% better and the vertigo improved. After the third treatment, all that was left was some of the vertigo.

There is a very good exercise for vertigo called the Epley Maneuver. It is easy and safe to learn, and for this patient was very useful. Her vertigo was resolved after the treatment.

Stubborn root canal

"Jack"

24 Yr old man came in with terrible tooth pain after a root canal had gotten infected. He had taken multiple rounds of antibiotics, and had suffered through 3 root canals on the same tooth. The pain was on a lower mid tooth, and he had a low grade fever for the last 2 months. I knew his immune system was compromised, which would need to be treated with herbs and diet, but the pain should be treatable with acupuncture.

We needled ST43 ipsilateral, and PC4-6 contralateral. LI4,3, ST36, and LI10 all bilateral. His pain was reduced 50% during the first treatment, and we sent him with herbs to treat infection as well as to boost the immune function. The herbs were pills and kept separate so he could adjust the dose as needed. If he felt less pain, he could take more of the immune boosting formula, and if he felt more infection, take more of the clear heat and toxin formula. We didn't want to tonify the infection.

With weekly treatment, he was pain free after one month, but it took three months to completely cure the infection.

Bleed Bell's

"Julie"

28 Yr old woman presented in the clinic with Bell's palsy. I had been teaching the week before in class about how great bleeding cupping was for acute Bell's palsy, and one of my students sent in a family member who contracted it the morning of the first treatment. What a great chance to treat such an acute symptom.

The left side of her face was effected, from the eye to the nose and the mouth. There was no muscle tone to speak of, and everything felt numb. For this condition I look along the ipsilateral leg at the image level for veins. Most of her symptoms were on the ST and LI channel, but some GB and BL at the eye as well.

I used a lancet to prick the veins I found from ST36 to ST38 and from GB34 to GB39. We then attached plastic disposable cups to the pricked areas and let them drain 3-5 minutes until the bleeding stopped. The points were then needled deeply, with LI4,3 bilateral. She came in daily for 4 days. After the first treatment, her eye was able to open and close. After the second treatment her mouth was getting some of its tone back and the eye looked normal. Following the third treatment, her mouth was nearly normal, but the nose would not wrinkle when she grimaced. The condition was completely resolved 2 days after the 4th treatment.

Neck

Tonsillitis

"Kathy"

64 Yr old woman entered the clinic with a terrible case of tonsillitis. She had pain with swallowing and talking, and her lymph were very swollen. It seemed a little worse on the left side. We needled right LI5, PC7, and bilateral KD5-3. Her pain reduced immediately 50%. We added ST41 and LI4 bilateral. Her lymph were less tender and the throat kept improving over the next 2 days. The second treatment resolved the pain and swelling. We gave her an herbal formula that clears heat and toxins to take as needed and to prevent recurrent infections since she was getting them yearly.

Cervical fracture

"Agnes"

82yr old woman presents with neck pain, stating she had fallen 6 months previously, broken c2 cleanly and had a screw installed surgically to repair. When she came in she was in constant 6-7/10 pain. Channels involved: GB, BL, GV, TW, SI, LI. She had very little range of motion in any direction and constant pain. She had an x-ray the week previous and was told the bone was not healing after 6 months and at her age it probably would not. We started with the protocol we like for most bilateral neck pain: R-L - HT4,6, LU7,9, SP5.5, LR5. This set treats most neck and upper back pain. HT points are needled from the SI side (like other distal point practitioners use), SP6 is low, more like SP5.5. LR5 is an area which can take 3 needles to cover. I like to needle from the crest of the tibia toward SP channel, tenting the skin and needling transversely. This set helped the pain 50% or better. We then added: Upright Tendon, alternating the side each treatment, and KD3-7 area for the LI channel pain on the scalene and scm. This is needled close to the Achilles tendon. Zheng Jin area is one of my favorite Master Tung points. Needled through the Achilles tendon to the back of the tibia. I like to divide the tendon into 7 parts from the start of the tendon at the end of the gastrocnemius (C7) to the insertion on the calcaneous (occiput). The depth of the needle depends on the problem. If the spine is tender, it is usually just the tendons and ligaments that are sore, so needling into the Achilles tendon is sufficient. If there is a bone problem, like a broken vertebra, then the needle needs to touch the bone, in this case the back of the tibia. In fact, we usually tap on the back of the tibia with the tip of the needle a few times each treatment. We also gave her various blood circulating and regeneration herbs in pill form.

These points relieved most of the pain each treatment. The pain did return after a few hours at first, then started lasting days after a few weeks of treatment. She received treatment 3-4 days per week. After 4 weeks her pain was minimal, 1-2/10, and not constant. Her range of motion seemed normal. A few weeks later she hit her head again and heard a crunching sound. She went to the ER for an x-ray and they confirmed everything was still in place and that the bone was healing and looked good.

Upper Back

Smokers back

"Jessi"

This 43 yr old woman presented with upper back pain in the rhomboids, levator scapula, and paraspinal muscles. We started treatment using the tried and true HT4-7, LU7-9, SP5.5, LR5. This set covers most channels on the upper back. Much of the pain would resolve, except for an area on the rhomboid muscles.

While looking at her hands we noticed many veins in the thenar eminence. We could also smell strong nicotine on her. She had been a smoker for over 20 yrs. After needling Chong Zi and Chong Xian, the pain would relieve for a few days, and it was not until we bled these points that she got lasting relief.

Subscap lessons
"Jeff"

39 Yr old man came in for treatment complaining of severe muscle pain is his upper back after painting his ceiling 2 days prior. After palpating around and not finding much pain in the usual suspects of trapezius, levator scapula, rhomboids, and paraspinal muscles, I wondered if it could be something deeper.

Treatment began with HT4, LU7, SP5.5, LR5, and Chong Zi – Chong Xian. The pain only relieved 20%, so I kept palpating distal points. He was also complaining of pain in the axila, which is HT1, so I needled KD3 and got 50% total relief. After palpating the axila it occurred to me that subscapularis was extremely tender. I started thinking about why KD3 helped so much, and decided to try treating HT channel for subscapularis. Opposite clock is GB, and at the upper back level, GB39. I started needling it in the traditional location at the posterior side of the fibula, but did not get much effect. I then tried the front of the fibula and was able to needle deeply to what I now know to be the interosseus membrane. After that point his pain was down to 10%, and his ROM was normal.

I like the idea that subscapularis is between the scapula and the ribs, and that this point is not only between the tibia and fibula, but also between extensors and flexors at the interosseus membrane. The subscapularis muscle is related to the iliacus on the pelvis, but it is hard to needle efficiently and this point works well.

Upper back rib pain
"Fred"

56 Yr old man came to the clinic complaining of upper back pain that he had for five years. After treating all the regular muscles with HT4-7, LU7-9, SP5.5, LR5, and

GB39, the pain was only reduced by 20%. After palpating around more, the front ribs were very tender at KD27-25 as well as CV22. I needled CV22 in front of the manubrium and the KD points in the front, and the pain was gone. Interesting there was no restricted breathing, and he had no idea the front of his chest was even tender. 5 treatments resolved his condition. I am not sure if the ribs were actually out of alignment, or just that the muscles were spasming around them.

Chiropractic rib

"Luke"

One of my students years ago was a bartender, and he came in with a very painful upper back. He said that he was lifting a bin of glassware out of the washer when he heard and felt a "pop". Within minutes he was in massive pain with respiration or movement of the upper back of any kind. He had gone to a chiropractor to have the rib put back in, but after they made the adjustment, the condition worsened. By the time he got to me, he was not moving his neck or torso much at all, and every breath was labored.

After palpating around, his scalene muscles, trapezius, and ribs 3-6 were very tender in the left side. I needled on the right; HT4,5,6, LU7, KD3-7x3, SP5.5, LR5, SP5/LR4. I also needled CV17-22 for pain on the GV spinous processes. On the left I needled ribs 3-6 on the chest at the sternal junction and obliquely at the intercostal spaces at 1 and 3 cun increments. He no longer had pain with respiration, and had 50% ROM of the neck. He left feeling much better. He came back after 2 days and got the same treatment. It had not worsened since the first treatment. The following day, after the second session, he was back to work. He said that when he went back into the same position that caused the "pop", he felt like someone had punched him in the back, and the pain was gone.

I think ribs and bones can adjust themselves if the muscles are relaxed enough. Even chiropractors will agree that if the muscles are too tight they cannot adjust. Relaxation of the muscles is the key, and we have one of the best methods that exists. Non invasive treatment, instant relaxation, pain relief, and increased blood flow are just a few of the benefits of distal acupuncture.

Low Back

12th inning

"Rosie"

62 Yr old woman complained of back pain that she was having trouble finding anything that worked for it. We were at a baseball party and I offered to treat her. She had tried acupuncture before, and it was usually effective for her, but the treatments were not helping this problem. After lying her on a couch, I palpated around and found a very tender spot on the left lateral attachments of the 12th rib.

I usually think of rib as GB and LR channels, but the 12th rib stops at the BL channel. I first needled LU5-6 on the contralateral right side, and BL57 on the ipsilateral left side. This helped 20%, so I added GB34 on the ipsilateral side. Now the pain was 30% better. I had treated BL and GB channels, so I tried treating LR channel with Gan Men yang area (see point description) on the contralateral right side. The pain was 50% better. There was an idea I had that the quadratus lumborum was involved with the 12th rib and belt channel, so I needled GB41 on the ipsilateral left side. The pain was now 80% better, and the baseball game had gone to 12 innings.

Experience has shown that this 12th rib is a crossing of belt, LR, GB, and BL channels. My current formula for this is contralateral LU5-6, Gan Men yang, and ipsilateral GB34, 41, BL57-40. GB41 works best when needled under the extensor tendon toward GB42.

"Sacroiliac joint point (SI Jt pt)"

This point was invented out of necessity. It is located 0.5" distal and medial to SI 6. Needled deeply to HT 7 if possible. Depending on the anatomy, this point when needled can start to come to the surface at SI 5 or near HT 7. It is very tight and sticky because the needle travels through a few of the ulnocarpal ligaments, and some patients have tight joints in their wrist.

This point location came about in a search for a point to treat the sacroiliac joint deeply. With the idea of like treating like in mind; muscles treat muscles, bones treat bones, skin treats skin, and tendon and ligament treat tendon and ligament. Just needle the tissue you need to treat. The gluteus maximus that originates along the lateral dorsal surface of the sacrum and over the sacroiliac joint, is treatable with muscle and tendon attachments. An area around TW 15 at the levator scapula insertion is effective. But it has not been effective for the deep sacroiliac joint pain that is ligamentous in nature. We need a joint and the ligaments in that joint for effective, consistent, predictable treatment. We would take advantage of the Ling Gu, Da Bai set, and add SI 4,5 to the treatment and would get mixed results with the sacroiliac pain.

One day I was treating a patient on a table that was up against a wall. I had to reach over the patient to needle SI 4,5 from an unseen angle. As I did, I got the angle off and the tip of the needle from SI 5 started to emerge at the surface near SI 6. The needle had travelled through the joint dorsally, puncturing ligaments and traveling under the tendon of flexor carpi ulnaris. Her sacroiliac pain was relieved immediately. We started playing around with needling this area from various locations, and finally found that the insertion from .5" distal to SI 6, toward HT 7 is most effective. The needle passes through 2-3 ligaments, and will relieve pain in the deep sacroiliac joint nearly every time. It does take some practice, and a thicker needle helps, though I now needle it with my preferred needle, a 1.5" 38ga. I feel free-handing this point is important as the window is so tight and it will take some force to get it through the ligaments.

Post postpartum lumbar strain

"Katie"

32 yr old patient presented with acute pain brought on 3 weeks after childbirth while lifting heavy objects. She came in with so much pain she was not able to lay on the table. We put her in a recliner, and started treatment. After palpating thoroughly, she was spasming all around the lumbar vertebra from L1-S1. The right sacroiliac joint was tender, the paraspinal muscles were extremely tight as was gluteus maximus. Psoas and QL were also involved on the right side.

I needled Ling Gu, Da Bai, SI3-4 on the left. After checking again, the pain was 50%, but in all the same areas. I then needled SI9-10 with 8 needles, BL58 area on both sides with 2 needles each, BL60, and KD3. Now her pain was mostly gone. The SI joint, thoracolumbar fascia at the SI joint, and lumbar spine at L4-S1 still had tenderness. I needled SI Jt Pt on the left, TW15 on the left, and CV4-6. Now her pain was less than 20%. Needles were retained 45 min. The pain continued to lessen and was completely resolved after 2 days.

Biker Butt

"Mel"

56Yr old woman presented with tailbone pain after taking a long motorcycle ride. The pain was located at the coccyx and to the right and left at the muscles that attach there. Top treats bottom, needle GV20 for GV1. I like to insert 2-4 needles in this area, angling them in a wedge shape. She also has digestive weakness and on hara palpation the zones that showed symptoms were SP center, LI right and left, ST, and LR lower left. We used the classic ST36, SP9, PC6 all bilateral, SP5/LR4 left sided. The coccyx pain was relieved immediately, and after 4 treatments resolved completely. Her digestive conditions are ongoing.

Hip

Piriformis syndrome

"Jackie"

A 36 Yr old woman presented with pain is her gluteus area after a long run. After palpating the areas thoroughly, the pain and tightness were located at gluteus maximus, medius, piriformis, obturator and gemellus. The piriformis was the most involved with pain at the sacrum attachment, muscle belly, and insertion at the trochanter. She was also having pain shooting down the sciatic nerve into her thigh.

I needled opposite shoulder SI9-10 area with 10 needles to cover the zone. I needled teres minor for piriformis, obturator and gemellus. Also, into infraspinatus and posterior deltoid for the gluteus muscles. Pain, ROM, and tension relieves quickly with these points and the condition resolved in 2 treatments.

Groin pain

"Jim"

67 Yr old gentleman presented with groin pain that radiated from the lateral hip, over ASIS, down inguinal ligament, and to the pubic tubercle. He had been suffering with this pain for 3 months and did not remember any specific injury.

ASIS relates with coracoid process and the pubic tubercle with the sternoclavicular joint. We needled the opposite LU1-2 and between the clavicle and the first rib into subclavius. We also needled around the sternoclavicular joint and KD27. Relief was immediate, and he could stand up straight again after the treatment. We treated him twice a week for three weeks at which time he was pain free.

Chest and Abdomen

PMS breast tenderness

"Gerry"

33 Yr old woman presented with PMS. The predominant symptom was breast tenderness, which she had continuously for over ten years, but got extremely painful around her menses. Her pain was on all the chest channels around the breasts, KD, ST, and PC.

We started with needling bilateral LI6-8 threading the 2 needles distally along the

LI channel, tenting the skin to assist with insertion. The pain reduced 30%, and was now mostly on the ST and PC channels. I then needled ST38-39 bilateral, and that reduced the pain another 20%. We added PC5-6 bilateral and the pain was now 85% better. We also needled LR3,4, LI4, SP6. She was also given herbs. After a series of 5 treatments the breast tenderness was no longer constant and only mild during the menses.

Fishing heart

"Paul"

54 Yr old man walked into the clinic complaining of chest pain. The first question I ask is have you been to a primary care? After he assures me they have done all they can for him, I take his blood pressure and it is 205/140! I am worried he will stroke out on my table. He is on every blood pressure medication I have ever heard of, and it is still that high. He fills me in on his history of severe drug abuse to the point of his heart failing and his blood pressure being out of control. "But I eat fish every day," he says. "That's why I am still alive." The scientific studies show otherwise, but I treat him anyway. Master Tung has a great set of points for physical heart conditions. They are located in a zone proximal to ST32 on the ST channel. I start needling three points in this zone, alternating sides each week, with PC6, ST36, GB40,41, LR3, Ling Gu, and GV20. His chest pain starts diminishing over a few months to the point he is able to fish and lay tile again for his job. His blood pressure came down some as well to 160/105. He continues to get treatment.

Construction shingles

"Gary"

Gary, a 34 Yr old man, presented with shingles pain in the classical hypochondriac region. He had been suffering with the nerve pain for 6 days and had not been able to work his construction job since the pain began. The skin was starting to break out, and when he came in he was making so much moaning noise that I stopped what I was doing with another patient and went straight to him. I asked where the pain was and he motioned to his left side and around to the back. I just inserted 3 needles in

LU6, HT3.5, and Gan Men yang area all contralateral. He started laughing. He never had acupuncture, was sent in by his father, and didn't believe it would do any good after all the pain pills he had tried with no effect.

After the needles were in for 30 min, he needed to go to the bathroom. We pulled the needles, and when he came back the pain had returned 50%. I put the 3 needles back in, and he stayed another 90 minutes. We never saw him again. His father said that he was so shocked about how well it worked that he thought it was some kind of magic, and that he had gone back to work the next day.

Psoas back pain
"Char"

55 Yr old woman presented with lumbar pain. On palpation the tenderness was more in the area of right sided quadratus lumborum and wrapping around to ASIS and psoas. My favorite points for psoas pain and tension are GB41 ipsilateral and pec minor contralateral.

We needled GB41 and the pain reduced 50%. We added pec minor points from LU1-PC1, and the pain was now 80% better. The pain completely resolved in 4 treatments.

Extremities

Scarred nerves
"Jose"

40 yr old Hispanic construction worker presented with hand numbness from injury. Jose came into the clinic with one of the most shocking scars I had ever seen.

During his construction job he had accidentally cut through most of his wrist with a hand held circulating saw. The channels cut were PC, LU, LI, and TW. The surgeons had done some great work reconnecting his hand tendons and ligaments, and amazingly he regained most of hand function. He did however have complete numbness from the scar to the thumb, index and middle fingers, palmar and dorsal.

We started needling the contralateral ankle and foot, covering it with dozens of needles, all name pair. We then came to find out that LR on the foot treats the dorsum of the hand, not PC. This led to comparative anatomy, and a study into contralateral correspondence.

Jose could actually feel the sensation coming back on various parts of his hands and fingers as we needled the related areas. He wouldn't even look at where we were on his foot, just run his other hand over the effected areas feeling for a change in sensation. In the beginning the effects from the acupuncture would wear off in a few hours, but as a few weeks went by, it took less needles to get the sensation back, and it lasted longer. By the time we had treated him for 3 months, there was only one numb area left around the scar itself, all the fingers had their sensation back.

He came back into the clinic after 3-4 months and reported that it had lasted for 2-3 months, then started getting numb again. After 1-2 weeks of further treatment, the numbness was again relieved.

After this case I started hypothesizing that nerves can have scars just like all other tissue, and these scars are like a kinked electrical wire, sending missed signals to the brain. As the distal treatments take effect, the brain starts paying more attention to the area effected by the needles, and gets more information, like increased sensation or reduced pain. That may also be why the effects are immediate. Blood circulation is most certainly increased, but the effect would not be instant if nerve were not somehow involved.

Thumb and wrist pain

"Jen"

42 yr old woman presented wrist pain L side, TW, LI, LU, around the thumb jt at LU9, LI5, and the tendon running between them. Pain on pressure from weight bearing on assisted raising from seated position. Pain came on gradually from repetitive injury, 4 weeks. Name Pairs are the best choice with the extremity image. The points 2x/wk were

Sp5x3, St41x2, and GB40x2, all on the R side. Pain reduced immediately, but with continuing the repetition of computer work, would return within a few days. After 2-3 weeks the pain was significantly improved. Then she went to see a chiropractor who adjusted the wrist joint, and aggravated the condition which took another 4 treatments to settle back down. This aggravation led me to think that the ligaments and tendons were involved which explains why the treatments were taking so long. She had complete pain relief after another month of treatment, and is still doing the repetitive work.

Phantom limb

"George"

54 yr old Caucasian veteran presented with fantom limb pain on his right foot. This patient came into the clinic in a wheelchair, and asked if we could help his phantom limb pain. When I asked him to describe the location and what feeling he was having, he looked at me as if I were joking. I guess no one had taken him seriously for his condition before.

He drew an area with his finger over the side of his intact foot on ST, GB and BL channels and said it felt like a horse was standing on it. We quickly needled the opposite hand between the 3rd and 4th metacarpals, TW3-4, and SI3-4. When asked how it now felt, he was shocked and said it felt like the horse got off his foot. The condition was resolved completely in 3 treatments.

This is another example of what I like to call nerve scarring. One might think that the scar would be at the stub of the leg near the knee, but the distal hand points still worked for the foot pain, even when there was no foot. I came to the conclusion that it must be brain correspondence we are working with.

Achilles heel

"Janet"

53yr old woman presented with Achilles tendon pain, R side, 2" proximal to the calcaneus. This patient used jogging as her main form of exercise. It would cause the tendon to become inflamed and painful with weight. We started using the opposite wrist on the ulnar tendon from HT4-7 with 50% improvement. These treatments were continuing 2x per week for 4 weeks, at which time the condition plateaued. There was 20-30% of the pain remaining. We then found that the ankle – neck relationship became the best alternative and finished the pain off in 2 treatments. The points were BL9-10 area, and extending down the BL channel with 3 needles. In addition points were needled along the cervical spine at the same level. I had found that GV20-16 was effective to treat the heel, but in extending the image, there is also effectiveness for the Achilles tendon (just like Zhong Jin treats the neck).

Singing heel pain

"Wind"

46 Yr old woman presented with heel pain after standing and singing at a gig she had a month previous. The pain was on both feet, mostly on the left. I usually try to differentiate the area of pain for foot and heel pain. Her pain was at the exact bottom center of the heel on both sides. We needled Mu guan and Gu Guan, altering the location slightly toward the pisiform bone which I believe is anatomically the calcaneus. Three needles total were inserted on the pisiform.

I had her stand up with the needles in and walk around to see if the pain had changed. The right foot was completely better, the left still had some pain, but it had moved to the front of the heel, slightly medial. I think the anatomical equivalent on the hand is just distal to PC7. After needling that point on the left, the right foot was resolved as well. The pain came back after 2 days, and she was treated twice a week for one month. The pain has not returned.

Weekend warrior knee

"Kent"

35 Yr old man came in experiencing swelling and pain in his right knee after a long weekend riding his bike. He had not been on it in over a year and overdid the exercise. The swelling was noticeable, and he had tightness inside the joint on flexion of

the knee.

I really like the Master Tung treatment for swelling of the knee. It is a circulatory treatment, and the image is difficult to figure out. Needle PC6 contralateral and LR3 ipsilateral. I have the patient flex and extend the knee for ten reps every ten minutes, kind of like "pumping" the fluid out of the joint. The effect is remarkable. By the end of the treatment, the swelling will be down by at least 50% and most of the time gone entirely. Two treatments resolved this knee pain.

References

Anatomy

Grey's Anatomy (35th British edition)
Warwick and Williams

Thieme Atlas of Anatomy – General anatomy and musculoskeletal system
Michael Schuenke M.D. Ph.D. and Erik Schulte M.D.

Thieme Atlas of Anatomy – Head and neuroanatomy
Ross, Lawrence M., M.D., Ph.D.

Rehabilitation

7 Steps to a pain-free life (updated edition)
Robin McKenzie with Craig Kubey

Advanced Tung Style Acupuncture
James H. Maher D.C., O.M.D., Dipl.Ac.

Acupuncture 1,2,3
Dr. Tan's Strategy of 12 Magical Points
Twelve and Twelve in Acupuncture
Twenty-Four More in Acupuncture
Richard Teh-fu Tan and Stephen Rush, OMD, Lac

Lectures on Tung's Acupuncture – Therapeutic System
Illustrated Tung's Acupuncture Points
Lectures on Tung's Acupuncture – Points Study
Tung's Acupuncture
Dr. Wei Chieh Young

Master Tung's Acupuncture – An ancient alternative style in modern clinical practice
Miriam Lee

A Guide to Su Jok Therapy
Jae Woo Park

A Manual of Acupuncture
Peter Deadman and Mazin Al-Khafiji with Kevin Baker

Nan-Ching – The Classic of Difficult Issues
Pien Ch'io
Translated by Paul U. Unschuld

Made in the USA
Lexington, KY
23 April 2018